FERTILE

Prepare Your Body, Mind, and Spirit for
Conception and Pregnancy to Create
a Conscious Child

PRITAM ATMA

ISBN: 978-0-578-53308-7

Printed in the United States of America

Table of Contents

DEDICATION

To You, a Divine Mother

"I am working to bring peace to the Earth — all we need is one kid and one womb and one woman and one man."

YOGI BHAJAN

APRIL 8, 1982

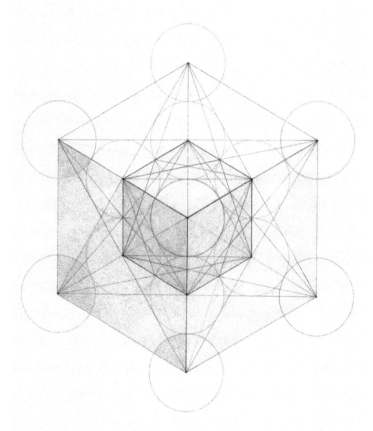

Metatron's Cube

ABOUT THE AUTHOR

Pritam Atma (previously named Chelsea Ann Wiley) wrote *Fertile* as part of a series and follow-up to her first book, *Mystical Motherhood: Create a Happy and Conscious Family a Guidebook for Conception, Pregnancy, Birth, and Beyond.* She is deeply connected to bringing conscious children into this world. She currently works as a Nurse Practitioner in a fertility center within the New York area, practicing Reproductive Medicine. Pritam Atma also works with women privately and in groups, helping them to apply the concepts of *Mystical Motherhood* and *Fertile* to increase their fertility and consciously prepare for motherhood. You can learn more about this at:

www.mysticalmotherhood.com

Facebook: Mystical Motherhood

Instagram: @mysticalmotherhood

She has also worked as a labor and delivery nurse at the top medical center: the University of California, San Francisco, and studied with Ina May Gaskin, the most famous midwife in the world. She is a board-certified Family Nurse Practitioner (FNP) and a Kundalini Yoga and Meditation teacher. At the hospital and in the primary care clinic, she found that families were unprepared for birth and parenting, that they lacked knowledge to maintain health, and yearned for a deeper understanding of how to integrate spiritual practices into daily life. Pritam Atma envisions raising the consciousness of families around the globe and changing the frequency of the women who bring children into this world so that the next generation can live as peaceful, vibrant, and healthy individuals. She wrote this book for mothers, as she is a mother herself and knows that this population will change the world as we know it.

About the Artist

Kate Serenity Savage is a classically trained fine artist, illustrator and creative consultant. She possesses the unique ability to translate ideas into a cohesive visual language and the skill to express the essential level of artistry. Her artistic expertise lies in substantiating modern ideas with aesthetic tradition and has a special eye and discernment for the ubiquitous humanist themes of classical mythology, persona archetypes and great traditional narratives. Kate's work is most significantly influenced by, but not limited to, the great nineteenth century naturalists, classical antiquity and vintage art nouveau and art deco. She can be found on Instagram at @kateserenitysavage or on her website at www.kateserenitysavage.com.

INTRODUCTION

There is an eternal quest within human beings to discover and attain the Holy Grail. Historical battles were fought to maintain power over it, the Knights Templar vowed to protect it, and religions across the planet have tried to disguise it within ceremony to keep it a secret. King Arthur coordinated great spiritual expeditions to search for a relic. The majority of individuals have no idea what it is, and believe it to be some sort of an object, because it has been hidden within the dark ages. Cultures disguised the Grail within fables, stories and myths. Most recently, *The Da Vinci Code*, movie and book, more accurately described the Grail by explaining that Mary Magdalene held the bloodline of Jesus Christ by conceiving and birthing a holy child with him.

The Holy Grail, or the sacred chalice, is blood held within form that holds Christ Consciousness DNA. This blood has a higher frequency—a frequency shared by the enlightened Beings that have walked our planet including Jesus, Buddha, Quan Yin, Mother Mary, and Mary Magdalene to name a few. These saints and sages walked through dark times lighting the way for others to follow. Now those ages have come to an end, and you are here to usher in the enlightened age of man by birthing a new type of child onto this planet. I will teach you how to become this sacred chalice so that you are able to hold this higher vibrational DNA within yourself and your womb.

You can do this by healing every aspect of your body, mind, and spirit through an interplay of clearing individual cells and memories that compose the holographic sacred geometrical architecture of your existence. This simply means that by changing your thoughts, beliefs, emotions, environment, and diet, you can change your life and baby. Science is now proving that DNA can be altered and programmed through a field called behavioral epigenetics. The purpose of *Fertile* is to merge science and Spirit so that you can create a new frequency within your genome and become capable of conceiving, creating, and birthing a higher caliber Being onto this planet. Woman, you are the Holy Grail.

This book is written for women who are struggling with fertility, want to consciously conceive, and those who are already pregnant. It is applicable to women who have no children and those who want more. The transformational process can be utilized whether you become pregnant naturally or with medical help from intrauterine insemination, in vitro fertilization or a donor egg. The concepts are so universal they can be easily applied to every age and gender, but are critical for women who have a mission of birthing a high-caliber child. I wrote this text specifically for women in the childbearing period because I know that the fastest way to create a new and better Earth is through birthing healthy and highly conscious children. We are on the verge of self-destruction, which is leading to massive world destruction. In order to change on a larger scale, we have to begin to look at all the details of our lives—our choices and our personal environments. I hope to show you that there is a different way to live and that you are not a victim, but rather a commander of your existence. My aim is to give you your power back as a woman because you birth the children onto this planet.

My educational background and working experience have provided me with an exceptional amount of insight into the Western medical system. As a Nurse Practitioner working at a fertility center, I witness firsthand the impact that infertility has on men's and women's lives. And when I worked as a labor and delivery nurse and Family Nurse Practitioner, I saw a huge gap in our patient care. The mental, emotional, and spiritual needs of pregnancy were not met and rarely acknowledged. Many of the patients I engaged with in the primary care setting were coming in as a result of loneliness, but were being provided with an antidepressant to meet their needs. And regarding the needs of the not-yet-born child, in my undergraduate studies, I majored in Psychology and memorized every child developmental theory there was. As far as I know, not one theory mentions the time in the womb as being a significant period of development beyond the physical characteristics of the child.

I now work with many women around the world who are struggling with infertility and are applying the concepts of my previous book, *Mystical Motherhood*, to their lives. The average Western practitioner tends to miss the emotional, mental, and spiritual aspects that affect fertility. I help women approach fertility holistically. Many of my private clients have achieved pregnancy naturally as a result, despite discouragement and doubt from the Western medical system. As a society, we have become so reliant on pharmaceuticals and technology that we have forgotten the power that we hold within ourselves. If you are struggling to become pregnant, I cannot promise you that this book will absolutely solve this, but *I can promise* that you will walk away a more conscious individual who is comfortable on your personal journey to motherhood.

Fertile is a theory that will create a new paradigm. My intention is to teach women around the world that their thoughts, emotions, beliefs, and diet affect and program their growing fetus during the time of pregnancy. I want women to understand how critical this period of development is. My goal is to create a movement where women become incredibly conscious of the environment of their growing baby, understanding that they can purposely create a brilliant child, free from the generational patterns and programs that they once faced. Together, we are going to create a new world—one birth at a time.

As a global society, we have made the collective assumption that the fetus, and even the embryo, are not conscious. But, how could the fetus be considered conscious when the majority of humans on the planet are not conscious themselves? People run their lives making absolutely no connection between their mind, body, or spirit. Individuals currently do not understand the extent to which their emotions, thoughts or environment affect their cells and health. Nor do women currently understand how improving these influences during the period of conception and birth could create an advanced human race. Yes, I said that. You have that power.

The vibrational frequency of a woman before conception and during pregnancy is critical because it programs the DNA and the child. The amount of outside environmental stressors, such as food or toxins, that pregnant women encounter is astonishing. You may argue that some of these experiences are out of their hands, and I partially agree with that, but there are many more things that are within our control than we realize.

We need to explore the nature of our internal environments, both on an individual level and on a mass scale. If women do not explore their beliefs, trauma, thoughts, insecurities, or familial history before they become pregnant (or clear these things during pregnancy), they will pass these generational patterns on to their children. These internal states can be just as toxic as anything in the external environment. As a result of this lack of consciousness, we continue to create a human race that has not developed emotionally or spiritually much beyond the time of cavemen.

As I am writing this, today is March 2, 2018. I am not sure how many women will read this, nor do I have an idea of the number of women who will understand or follow through with the recommendations that are put forth within this book. I have a belief that the missing link to creating an awakened society lies within the womb of each woman who chooses to birth a child into this world in a conscious manner. I may not be alive to see if your children end up being more aware than the last generation. I guess I will never know if this theory is correct, which humbles me. In this moment, all I have is the power of my belief in your capability to birth a highly advanced child by altering your internal and external environments. What I am about to teach you about the power of the mind, body, and spirit makes this theory tangible and attainable. Because of that, I have hope that all of you are going to save this planet.

MERGING SPIRIT AND SCIENCE

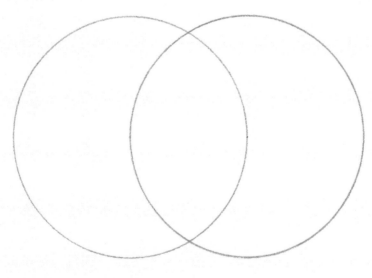

vesica pisers

CHAPTER 1

SPIRIT

The Fertility of Planet Earth

Mother Earth provides the best example we have of fertility. At her best, she creates life in ample abundance and flows forth everything needed for others to prosper. She magnifies the words lush, prosperity, wealth, health, reproduction, and elegance. She has the power to create Heaven within her body. Her ability to provide for her children makes this planet one of the greatest examples of motherhood that we have. The only thing that can impinge on her fertility is when her natural cycles are distorted from pollution, oil spills or taking too much of her life force. I am hoping that you can begin to see your own fertility process in a similar way that you experience the nature of Earth.

To understand this fully, I want you to imagine that you are now in your favorite natural area walking barefoot outside. Perhaps it is a park, lake, or hiking trail in the woods. Close your eyes and go to this place now. What does the energy in your body feel like walking here? What season is it and what are the colors that appear? Can you hear water flowing nearby or in the distance? Do you feel the heat of the sun, a breeze on your body, the earth under your feet? What scents come to you? Engage all of your senses and a heightened state of love and expansion within. Begin to experience it fully in the present moment. Sip in the experience like a slow inhale. Send your loving energy down into the earth of this sacred region so that the Earth can send her love back to you. Keep a note of this place so that you can always return to it. What would you want to emulate in yourself from this natural place that would create a fuller expression of your femininity? Perhaps it is the silence, colors, peace, smells, feeling of expansion, or sounds.

I am practicing this visualization right along with you and have many places on Earth that I can think of that I love to walk through, such as the mountains of Utah or the redwood forests of California. As I am writing this, I am in the natural landscape of Glastonbury, England, also known as Avalon. I would like to use this location as an example so that you can begin to emulate this type of abundant fertility within yourself. Avalon is a unique part of the world as it carries a significant amount of power within the land. Earth ley lines cross water ley lines creating a powerful vortex of energy which is palpable in the air and within the body. Avalon is the land of mystics and miracles. It is the representation of the Goddess here on Earth. The area defines lush fertility because the Shakti or Kundalini life force runs through it and helps it to produce beauty in abundance.

Hold my hand and imagine yourself walking through the countryside along-side me. Together, we open a gate to descend a path in the middle of two fields. Engage all your senses through this process. The energy is electric and the area is alive. The mists of Avalon create tangible veils which you can push to the side in your mind's eye as you walk through the fields. Moving these veils reveals hidden realities that go deep into the ground and extend far into the sky creating a sense of Heaven on Earth. All of your senses become heightened and you can literally feel, hear, taste, see and fully experience creation at its peak. You begin to understand that the reason that this land is so fertile and alive with life is because it holds a tremendous amount of energy and light. This higher frequency begins pulsing through your body with the purpose of vibrating and uplifting every cell. As your world subtly mingles with the unknown, you don't know where you end and nature begins.

Let's continue to walk together so you can experience the fertility of Mother Earth through my words. It is Springtime in Avalon. One field merges into the next and you enter an apple orchard full of rows and rows of pink blossoming trees. Just like you, they are ready to bear fruit as an offering for all. These trees have stood steady as the winds from the mighty northern seas blew through and created a freeze across the land. They have felt the chill of life, but still thrive. Begin to connect to these trees and visualize the blossoms. The colors are vibrant and there is a pulsing of pink, white, green, lavender, brown, and red all around you.

Feel the vibration coming off the plant life combined with the textures of the grass and ground under your feet. Listen to the sounds as you walk. The birds sing in toned waves through the distance. Occasionally the wind blows, creating a new sensation and you can hear this tingle like soft bells as leaves speak through the trees. Springtime smells, such as jasmine or green grass, catch your attention. If you could taste them, they might be like fresh lemonade or sweet tea. You can feel the Goddess here because this is her land. You are in the womb of planet Earth and there is a feeling of total expansion and connection to divinity. When you become one with God or the Goddess like this, how could you not create the same thing inside of you? This is fertility.

Your greatest example of how to create life can be found in the abundance of nature around you. Yet we live disconnected from this experience because we use artificial light and have replaced fire with microwaves. We no longer walk in nature or gather our own food. This disconnection from the Earth is a disconnection from ourselves. If you want to increase your fertility, you must become like Springtime in Avalon and vibrate with life like the apple trees ready to bear their fruit. If you can create this lush fertile landscape inside of you—or at least the elemental balance, feelings, senses, and emotions that are connected to it—you will conceive and birth a vibrant soul. As you will soon learn, all of your senses and the elements of nature are involved in the process of conception and creation. Amplifying these can change your life and your children's.

Now let us think about a scene that does not hold this type of energy so you can understand what infertility might look like from Earth's point of view. Imagine you are in a busy section of a populated city. You begin walking through a bad part of town under a large highway. The rushing cars above create turbulent sounds and a shaky vibration, making you feel uneasy. Everywhere you look the only thing that you see is concrete. There are no trees because they wouldn't be able to grow through the physical density in this overdeveloped area. There are tents belonging to the homeless in the corners attempting to create shelter from the elements. The sounds make you incredibly alert. The rushing cars above, combined with the crunch of broken glass under your feet overwhelm your nervous system. All you can smell is car exhaust and trash, which leave a really strong fried chicken taste in your mouth. It doesn't feel good to be here. In fact, it feels isolating and scary. You begin to walk faster because your flight or fight response has turned on to signal that something is wrong.

This scene represents much of the Western World as we know it. It also depicts many individuals' inner landscapes as much as the outer ones that have taken up the natural settings around our planet. Fertility is a "sensual" experience. Nature provides the best example for you to emulate. She is your greatest teacher when it comes to conception, pregnancy, birth, and motherhood. My goal is to get your vibration so high that you become a walking Goddess representing Avalon in New York City. This is possible, but it is an inside job which requires a desire to become an awakened woman.

The Awakened Human

An awakened human being has a fully engaged sensory system, much like the frequency of Earth in full bloom. This creates an incredible peace and connection to the world around them. There are six senses that can be amplified: vision, hearing, taste, smell, touch, and proprioception (extrasensory perception: the relation to the body within its field). Similar to genes within your DNA, these senses can be turned on like a light switch. Individuals engage their senses in different ways. You can choose to eat average food, repeat the same experiences daily, play out dramatic relationships, carry negative thoughts, listen to foul music and watch violent TV. Or you could eat food that is nutritious and invigorating, listen to music that positively engages your nervous system and create outstanding and heart-opening experiences that expand your world. The person who chooses the latter carries a higher frequency. She would have an entirely different human experience than the first person and is likely highly connected to herself, her purpose and divinity. She is on the road to becoming an awakened human.

The greatest shift in perception I ever had, and the first time I ever felt any of this, was in my basement in 2012. I was having a "dark night of the soul" year and physically felt dense, lost and desperate. I had bought a book that had the word "Kundalini" in the title and sat down to repeat a mantra that I had randomly found while flipping through the pages. I had never meditated before, but all of the sudden a force larger than life began to pulse up my spine entering every region of my body, making me scream, laugh, cry, and shake uncontrollably. I heard the words "be grateful" softly spoken from a higher force. The only guidance I had as to what was happening to me was the book I had in front of me which discussed what a Kundalini opening actually was. The experience lasted around five hours and altered every cell in my body. I had no idea at the time that my life would never be the same, but I did know that all my senses had changed immediately. I became fully alive.

After this experience, my entire world became enhanced. My vision changed. Trees and individuals began to show halos of energy. I was also very sensitive and could no longer watch television or eat certain foods for a period of time. I had a tremendous amount of energy flowing through me, which needed to be dispelled by running or spending time in nature. I experienced more miraculous openings as years passed, and became clairvoyant and clairaudient as a result. A Kundalini rising creates a deep and persistent desire to know that you and God are one. This is self-realization. You can create this connection within yourself through meditation and mantras, something I discussed in much more detail in my first book, *Mystical Motherhood*.

When this particular experience happened, I had enough sense to keep my head on straight and use the situation to create a better version of my life. This entailed going deep into my subconscious and removing generational patterns, deep wounds, negative belief systems, emotions, and thoughts. Anything that separated me from Source, or Spirit, had to be eliminated. The Kundalini energy compelled me to keep healing every aspect of my mind, body, and spirit. This is the type of in-depth work I am going to teach you how to complete in this book. I am sharing my own story of awakening so you can see what is possible and also understand why and how I came to write this for you. My intention is to help you through your own spiritual growth so you can create a better world and awaken humanity through the children that you birth.

When an individual "awakens," their senses become enhanced and they literally see, taste, and feel differently. They begin to become attracted to higher experiences that match their own vibration, carefully choosing to be around positive people and healthy food because they literally can't attract anything less. They also choose better thoughts, beliefs, and emotions. An awakened individual has a highly different experience of their surrounding world than the average person. They attract opportunities and have a deep connection to Spirit. These higher vibrational Beings have increased intuition, joy and abundance because they carry more light, which might make them glow. You can see it in their eyes and on their skin. There are not that many of them, but if you are reading this, then I promise more are coming.

An unawakened individual has a much denser physical experience on Earth and could be compared to the street scene I mentioned earlier. Contrary to a "lighter" individual, an unawakened person has beliefs, thoughts, emotions and a diet that create more physical, emotional and spiritual density. You can see this in their health and the way that they approach life. Most of their experiences are the same day to day, and relationships are difficult. There is no time for creativity, expression or abundance because negative emotions or base needs take all of their energy. They are so caught up in their physical Earthly experience—of trauma and drama—that they would not be able to create greater expressions or serve others in a higher way. Their ability to "sense" is not as heightened and as a result, they will be more attracted to heavy music, violence, hate, pain, fast food, and negative relationships that play on repeat.

If you comprehend the senses, you can understand what makes Earth unique. Let's just pretend that you are on another planet or within another dimension, where the frequency is lighter and more vibrant, and as a result the "bodies" of the Beings are too. (Stick with me, yes, this is possible.) These ethereal Beings have fully engaged sensory systems that allow them to see and speak in telepathic ways that most individuals on Earth could not comprehend. As you drop down into the earthly plane, or the three-dimensional experience, bodies and human experiences are much denser. In order for you to attract an ethereal and light-filled soul from these higher planes of existence, and actually hold the child in your body, you must begin to match their frequency.

The Infertility Crisis

I believe this work is more important than we can currently understand. The rate of infertility is expected to rise up to fifty percent in the next forty years.[1] Perhaps you are dealing with issues around becoming pregnant now, or you know someone who is. With the exception of the women that are suffering, no one else is paying much attention to this, other than the big pharmaceutical companies or fertility specialists. I have personally worked with women all over the world, helping them improve their fertility by changing their thoughts, emotions, environment, and diet. These also happen to be the factors that affect your genome. When doctors did not know how to help these women, somehow this work did, and I hope it can do the same for you.

There are many theories as to why infertility occurs in women and men with no medical problems, such as environmental toxins, drugs and alcohol, pharmaceuticals, pollution or having children at an older age. What most of these things have in common is that they create density within humans, dulling the vibration of their cells. We have swiftly moved into the Age of Aquarius, which is also known as the Golden Age of man. Evolution is natural, and in order for a planet to create a higher species, only those with the best DNA would be able to reproduce. My theory, and I want to express again that this is just a theory, is that infertility is on the rise because the higher caliber Beings that want to come to Earth can only be birthed through women who carry the same frequency. They cannot make it through the density found in unawakened humans. There are currently not that many women on the planet who have done the work needed to clear the density, but there is hope now.

You will soon learn that what we once thought about genetics is not true. You are in control of your destiny and those of your children. Individuals with

---

1   (William, 2016)

enhanced DNA are higher functioning, carry a high-quality frequency, and have a heightened sensory system —all of which complement a lighter or more ethereal soul at conception. Before we dive into how to improve your body, mind, and spirit—in order to enhance your genome—you must understand why this is important at conception and how sacred geometry is connected to all of life.

Sacred Geometry and the Building Blocks of Life

At the moment of conception your frequency, or vibrational quality, determines the type of child that you will birth into this world. This sacred event involves all the senses of human existence here on Earth. You carry a specific vibration, sound, smell, feeling and taste which are unique to you and help to create your offspring. You also carry all the memories and karma of past generations within your cells along with your own unique destiny to potentially fulfill within your lifetime.

Sacred geometrical shapes are produced in a perfectly calculated mathematical order as an embryo develops, and this series of events is consciousness at its best. Consider your womb to be equal to the Void within all time and space. You are then the Universe within the Universe creating life for the All in absolute perfect harmony. The geometrical shapes created within your womb after conception and throughout pregnancy compose the basic building blocks of life, just like DNA. Each shape is deeply connected to an element found in nature such as fire, water, air, earth or ether. The geometry that unfolds within your womb from conception through pregnancy represents specific aspects of your being and facets of your generational history, physical existence, thought patterns, belief systems, and connection to Spirit.

This geometrical unfoldment of an embryo is the same sequence for all individuals on Earth and every living existence known to man. It ultimately creates the flower of life and the Fibonacci sequence, that can also be found within the details of a pine cone, a shell and a strand of DNA. If this sequence is always the same, why are humans fundamentally different? The variances within humans comes from the physical, mental, emotional, and spiritual state of the mother at the time of conception and during pregnancy. These various states of existence alter the DNA, making each individual unique.

The three basic shapes of the square or cube, the triangle or pyramid, and the circle or flower of life, all help to create the composition of the baby as cells divide within the womb to produce the fetus. This sacred geometry is also connected, in the same order, to the body, mind, and spirit. *Fertile* is broken up into these three sections to simplify the process of altering and improving each aspect of yourself before conception and during pregnancy with the intention of increasing your frequency so that you can produce an enlightened Being. We will dive deep into your various characteristics so that we can upgrade you before motherhood.

The purpose of this book is to help you clear your historical density from your bloodline so that you can attract a crystalline soul. Assuming that children choose their parents, this type of soul has no or few karmic links to the planet and selects parents according to their light quotient and vibrational frequency. When children like this are born, they will not have to spend the majority of their lives working through the personal problems, familial issues, wounds or attachments which are typically created from past bloodlines or previous lifetimes. Essentially, these children will be clear from the past because you have done the work to clear yourself. You can think of them as disconnected from cultural or societal belief systems that may hold them back in life. These children will be able to complete great missions or achievements to help this Earth to thrive without the personal resistance or self-sabotage that the typical human faces as a result of their energetic and genetic makeup.

It is my goal to help you improve your genome before conception and during pregnancy by holding up a mirror so that you can find your true self and improve your internal and external environment. Doing this will allow you to find all the joyous and beautiful parts of your soul that are connected to Source that you would like to pass on to your child. It will also help you identify all the ways that you can be neurotic, reactive, judgmental, angry, insecure, and depressed. You will be able to identify both why you act like this and the belief systems or thoughts that hold these emotions in place.

It is not necessary for you to pass these traits on to your children. This work isn't for the fainthearted or unmotivated. This is for women who are ready to face themselves and rise up. The ones who are committed to making an impact in their world. Birthing and raising conscious children is one of the most sacred acts you can do for this planet. There is tremendous amount of potential in the children of our future.

A Note to the Reader

Throughout the book I have included questions for you to answer, starting with the visualization below. In the future, I will have a workbook for you to dive deeper into the process of awakening. For now, please record your answers in the empty spaces within this book or keep a diary close. Recording your progress will keep you accountable for your own self-development. When you answer questions within *Fertile*, close your eyes and write down the first vision or thought that you have. Do not second guess yourself because intuition happens in the first seven to eleven seconds of thought. Recording your answers will enable you to see how you have changed over the course of exploring yourself through this book. It is your personal record of how you created a new frequency and ultimately changed your life for your babies.

The Moment of Conception:
The Visualization to Create an Enlightened Child

The following description of conception was communicated to me by a higher source and I will attempt to describe it to you as best I can through words. As you read the following visualization, picture the event of conception in your mind as it is described below. Become the woman on the bed who is about to conceive a child. I want you to do this so that you have a general sense of your current frequency. Understanding your vibration will give you a grasp of the energetics of conception and help you to see and feel the type of child you would currently attract, or have already conceived if you are currently pregnant. The moment of conception creates the base frequency for the type of soul you can carry. Begin to see, hear, feel, taste, and touch the experience of what happens within you and the cosmos when you decide to have a baby.

Begin by imagining yourself lying on a bed, knowing that you are about to conceive a child. Visualize an iridescent heavenly, soft, white light streaming down at an angle towards your womb. The column of light pours forth to Earth from the heavenly realms similar to that which you might see in a painting of a saint when he or she is being blessed from above. Visualize light drifting like soft, faint, wooly clouds with floating bright energetic flickers of light which look like stars. The symbol of the dove may appear as the energy moves slowly towards your body.

Touch

Though this light is soft and illuminating, it is also fierce and potent with energy. If you could touch this experience, it would have the texture of the type of soul you are going to bring in, which could range from angelic soft light to a thicker cloudlike material that brushes between the space of your fingers:

When you picture this energy entering into the room what does it immediately feel and look like? Do you see a texture or a color? If you could touch the energy with your fingers would it feel electric, magnetic, heavy, or light? Please describe it in detail and write down the first things that you see and feel.

As this spiritual energy moves closer to your womb, hovering approximately one to two feet above you, it pauses in time. Then, in a split second, it moves faster than the speed of light, entering your womb with a tremendous amount of power, like an arrow would hit a target directly on point.

Sound

When this spiritual photonic light energy merges with the womb, or when the sperm enters the egg, a sound resonates within the cosmos. A resounding vibration echoes through all of time and space as this holy event occurs. This is the sound frequency of your child.

If this were to happen at this moment in time, what would you hear? This sacred sound reverberation may be similar to a brilliant buzzing or to a thunderous Ommm. You may hear a Raaa, Maaa, Saaa, Taaa, Naaa or Maaa, or a combination of these sounds. Only you can hear this. Listen to the sound within yourself that is unique to you and write this down.

The potency and purity of the sound of creation produced within your child is dependent upon your sound frequency at the time of conception. As this sound of creation booms across the Universe, the angels may pause to smile because this is the reverberation of life forming. Beings may bow to your existence because within all of the cosmos you are completing one of the most sacred acts of receiving.

Sight

Now, imagine light shining out from the blackness of your womb. This light represents Source or consciousness and is a replica of what happens within the blackness of the cosmos at the time of Creation. Visualize this light as extensions of consciousness emerging out in six directions. These light beams are linear and have the potential to create basic geometric shapes. These beams emerge from the embryo within your womb which has just been fertilized. This represents the first signs of consciousness within you. Visualize this sphere, the embryo. The light will create an appearance on its surface. The shape of this circle is always the same, but the surface will appear different for each individual.

What does the consistency of the inner sphere or membrane look like? Is it buoyant like a trampoline? Does it look fragile, weak, thick or lacking energy? Does the sphere maintain its shape or is it flexible? Is it vibrant, smooth or rough?

The purer your connection to Spirit at the time of conception, the purer the frequency of this sphere or embryo. The higher your connection to the spiritual realms and the clearer you are, the stronger and more vibrant this surface will appear. The strength and perfection of this sphere at the time of conception is relevant because it forms the base level of consciousness of your child.

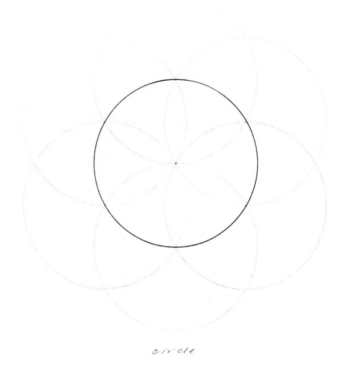

circle

Smell

Look within the sphere and you will see two small circles overlapping in-side forming what is called the vesica piscis. These two circles overlap in exact proportions with a region in the middle similar to the eye of the needle. This is the representation of the female and the male aspects of creation, each holding twenty-three chromosomes. In science, this event is referred to as the appearance of two pronuclei inside the egg demonstrating that fertilization has occurred, or that the sperm has entered the egg. The sphere or egg is now an embryo. Each circle of the vesica piscis has a smell, a scent from the male and a scent from the female. If you were to take an imaginary dropper and energetically place a scent into the two circles inside the embryo, what would you smell?

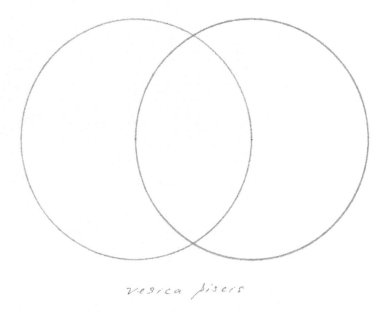

vesica pisers

What two smells represent these two circles? At the time of writing this, the scents that come to mind for me are those of purple lilacs and gardenias. Other scents could be frankincense, myrrh, rose, lemon, sandalwood, fresh grass, pine or even peaches. Other words you might use to describe these smells are: fruity, oceanic, woody, citrus, floral or spicy. You may be able to sense what two smells would create the makeup of your child if you were to conceive today. What are the first scents that come to mind? Even if they are not the most pleasant scents, please write them down.

Taste

The sacred geometry of the flower of life begins to form energetically within the embryo from these male and female aspects of creation. Identical spheres are repeatedly created outwards from the central point of the vesica piscis within the embryo. In your mind's eye, watch as the flower of life unfolds. Each new sphere is created in a delicate process, like a flower in bloom. The flower of life is a living map of creation—not just for your child but for all of reality as we know it.[2] As each sphere forms in the flower of life imagine that you are adding tiny droplets of liquid into each of the circles—individually creating flavors. What is the taste of these droplets of liquid?

What would this experience taste like if it were to happen to you now? You may be able to taste the type of child you are creating. As the process of creation continues, and each circle within the flower of life forms, there are various flavors that the child could be composed of including salty, spicy, sweet, sour, bitter or savory—or a combination of these. Your taste at the moment of conception will help to determine your child's makeup. Write these scents down.

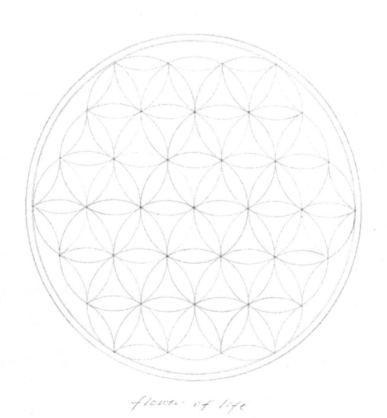

flower of life

---

2   (Melchizedek, 1998)

The flower of life is what creates consciousness and represents the develop-ment of Spirit within your womb. It is how God creates throughout the Universe. The entire process described above is only what occurs at conception, when the sperm enters the egg to unite, combine and form forty-six chromosomes. In Re-productive Medicine this is considered day one of embryonic development. As you can see, your sense of awareness plays a vital role, and your taste, smell, sound, sight, and touch all contribute to create the base frequency of your child. These are also sensational experiences that are heightened in nature and amplified within an awakened human being.

After this, the embryo begins to divide into two cells, then four, then eight, six-teen and onwards. The formation of these cells creates sacred geometric shapes within your womb. These geometric shapes match the frequency of elements found in nature. Understanding and exploring the characteristics of fire, water, earth, air and ether is the basis of *Fertile*. It will help you to create an enlight-ened child and will also allow you to comprehend the spiritual nature of the entire Universe.

The Sacred Geometrical Unfoldment of a Fetus

As the original embryo duplicates within the first few days after conception, all of the platonic solids are created within your womb. These include the cube, tetrahedron, octahedron, dodecahedron, and icosahedron. I have included drawings of all of this sacred geometry within *Fertile* and you will have a clearer understanding of the meanings of these shapes as you continue to read. These sacred geometrical shapes are linked to the elements which create the physical, emotional, mental, and spiritual makeup of humans. You may notice that I re-peat points throughout the book especially regarding sacred geometry and the elements. Drawings may be displayed twice. This is done intentionally. I hope to simplify complex subjects so that you can actually make concrete changes with-in your life. This knowledge will help you to balance your internal elements, affect the geometric configuration of your child, and change the makeup of the cells and genome.

Square or Cube

As the embryo begins to divide, the first platonic solid formed within the womb is the cube, which represents the composition of the physical body. The cube will energetically appear as dense or ethereal, depending upon the consciousness of the mother at the time of conception. The lighter or clearer the geometric shape is, the fewer generational or historical patterns the woman has left to let go of. Memories or karmic residue from the past create density held within the physical body. A person able to hold light or energy will not be physically constrained by drama, trauma or even food. A woman who works to clear her generational history, pain, sexual abuse or any memories held within the physical body will ultimately create a higher vibrational frequency. She will then attract and create a similar soul.

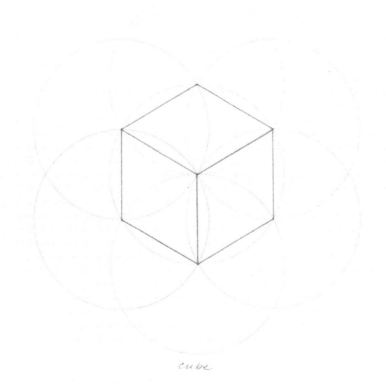

cube

If you close your eyes now what does your cube look like? Does it have a color or texture? Is it dark or light in color? Does it feel heavy in weight? Does it appear to be transparent or dense? Write down whatever comes to mind.

The cube contains eight cells which form what is referred to as the Egg of Life in sacred geometry. The Egg of Life is shown below as a three-dimensional drawing. You have to imagine that the eighth cell is hidden behind the others. In Reproductive Medicine this should appear on day three after fertilization. The frequency of this original shape is vital because it creates the basis of all of life. In the Body section of *Fertile,* I teach you how to create an ethereal Egg of Life, or lighter physical body, by altering your diet and healing your past.

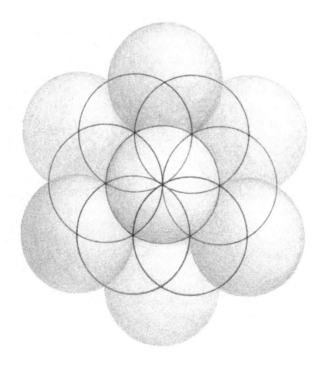

egg of life

The Triangle Pyramid or Tetrahedron

As the fetus continues to develop, two pyramids or tetrahedrons are produced. If you look at this in a different way, tetrahedrons also produce the shape of the cube. A triangle, or pyramid, represents the Holy Trinity within your womb. It solidifies your connection to the mind, body, and spirit or father, mother, and child. It is the shape that holds the power for ascension or resurrection on this Earth. It creates the Universal primal numbers of three, six, and nine. As the fetus develops, one pyramid is created and a replication of another pyramid develops on the opposite end, representing the saying "that which is above is that which is below." The Mind section of *Fertile* will help you become the Holy Trinity and connect to Spirit through your thoughts and relationship.

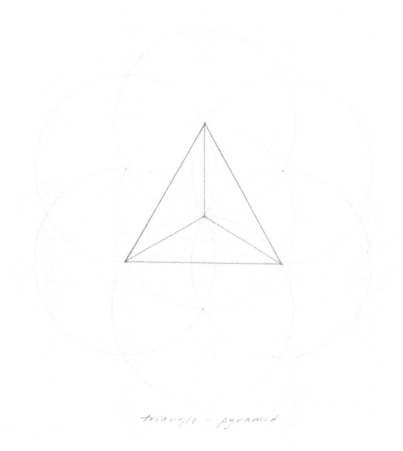

triangle - pyramid

The Platonic Solids

Fertile is purposely divided into the body, mind, and spirit in order to help you heal each of these aspects of your life. These sections also coincide with the labels of square, triangle and circle. These basic shapes help to form the platonic solids which create the base frequency of your child. If you heal the body, mind, and spirit aspects of yourself you will also clear the geometry of your baby. The platonic solids are energetically formed within your womb through embryonic development, and each geometric shape represents an aspect of the elements fire, earth, water, air and ether. It is important to have these elements in balance at the time of conception and during pregnancy in order to create harmony within your child. This will all be tied together in the Spirit section of the book.

Messages from Source

The information received above regarding conception and embryonic development was provided to me from a higher source through internal visions and descriptions. You could say that I entered the experience with the "no-mind", meaning I was completely open-minded and had no references or opinions on sacred geometry. I filled in a few details regarding the days of cell division from what I know as a result of working in Reproductive Medicine. Obviously, there is a lot more that needs to be included when you have zero understanding of a new concept. When I am in need of further knowledge, Source always sends me what I require next through a book or person. This helps to verify what I have learned and provide more information on how to utilize it. Before I go further into describing the geometrical creation of your baby, I want you to have a brief understanding of how most of the information in this book came together.

When I receive from Source, it is usually during meditation within clear visions that I can see and hear. When this happens, I am usually skeptical and a little shocked. I wish I wasn't, but it keeps me humble and in awe of just how powerful the Universe is. I relish getting verification of information, which usually comes through books or direct feedback from individuals after the fact. These are beautiful aha moments where grace comes in. I like to merge my scientific and spiritual aspects to find the truth. After receiving the knowledge described above, I received a book that verified many details that I described to you. This is how this entire book was written—an internal and external dance with Reality that I received while traveling to many sacred sites throughout the world.

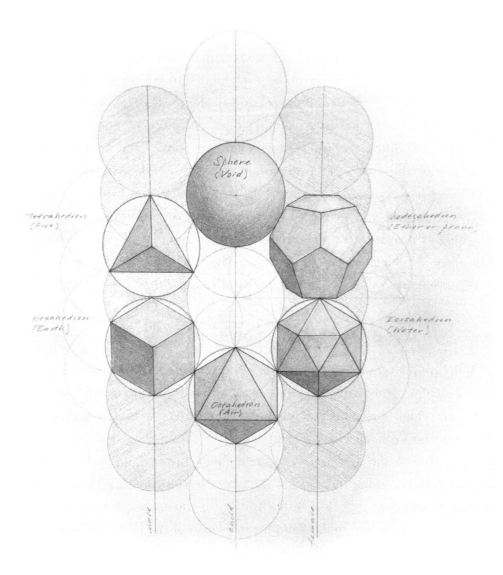

Spirit took profound steps to provide you this wisdom and if you are reading this now it is absolutely not a coincidence. The material I received to write this book (auditory, visual, books, and interviews) came to me in a myriad of ways that are almost unbelievable to the human mind. The purpose of this was to help you better understand how important your role is as a mother on this planet. Let me continue to explain what I received within this specific experience and then compare it to outside sources so that you can have a larger picture of how Spirit is deeply embedded in the process of creation.

Drunvalo Melchizedek wrote a book entitled *The Ancient Secret of the Flower of Life*. In Volume 1 of his series, he explained some of what I discussed above, but with a much more mathematical and in-depth description. His description of the information I received wouldn't have made much sense if I hadn't fully "experienced" it first. Sacred geometry can be complex and hard to understand. Melchizedek did a very good job summing up the entire Universe in his book and I highly recommend reading it if you are interested in understanding the full creation process in detail. I will summarize the important information for you here as it relates to conception and sacred geometry. I hope to break down complicated subjects within the worlds of Spirit and science and make them easy to comprehend so that you can actually utilize these theories in your daily life.

Spirit

Melchizedek summarized the cell replication process by explaining, "…we start out as a sphere, the ovum. We then move to a tetrahedron at four cells, then on to two interlocked tetrahedrons (a star tetrahedron or a cube) at eight cells. From two cubes at sixteen cells we turn back into a sphere beginning at thirty-two cells…." He was the first person to write about this and the flower of life which was previously hidden throughout the ages. He confirmed the vision I received that the flower of life can be found within the ovum and explained that the flower of life should have two lines around it to represent the inner and outer circle of the zona pellucida, or the membrane of the ovum. These two lines help to create an almost perfect phi ratio within the geometry, which is the basis of the golden ratio and mathematical equations found in all of nature including DNA.

Body

Melchizedek also described something called the Egg of Life, which is made up of eight spheres. He said, "Your entire physical existence is dependent upon your Egg of Life structure. Everything about you was created through the Egg of Life form, right down to the color of your eyes, the shape of your nose, how long your fingers are and everything else. It's all based on this one form." This is very important to note because the Egg of Life geometrically creates the cube which is the representation of the physical body. These original eight cells are identical in nature. This stage of development is critical because the energetics of these eight cells make up your entire structure.

He explained that these eight cells can still be found in their original form near your perineum. In the meditation, I asked you to record the density of the cube that you pictured in your mind's eye. The cube, or these original eight cells, is the closest thing to your true nature or original form that still exists within you. Our true nature is ethereal, but as life comes down to Earth, the original eight cells will become clouded by the density of the generational history, memories and physical characteristics which reside within the mother at conception. We will work on clearing all the parts of your physical body as we move through this book.

Mind

If you connect the spheres of cells within the Egg of Life with lines, Metatron's Cube is produced. Metatron's Cube holds the five platonic solids which are made up of unique geometrical shapes produced from cubes and triangles or pyramids. All of the elements are held within this unique geometry. Each of these shapes, together, make up who you are. In order for you to attract a high-frequency child, your elements need to be balanced and your thought forms should be free from negativity and outdated belief systems.

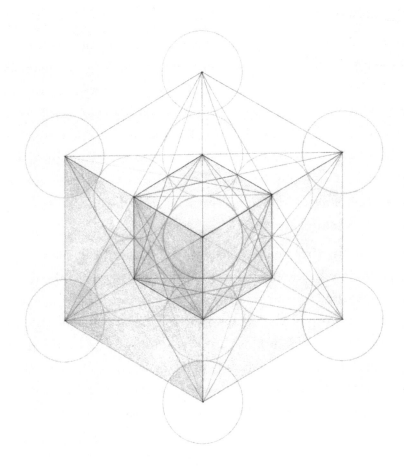

The five platonic solids held within Metatron's Cube are:

♣ Hexahedron or Cube (six sides with equilateral squares)—represents earth and is male energy

♣ Tetrahedron (three-sided pyramid)—represents fire and is male energy

♣ Octahedron (eight sides with equilateral triangles on each side)—represents air and the child

♣ Icosahedron (twenty faces of equilateral triangles)—the blueprint of life—contains the parameters of DNA and represents the element of water and the female. This shape is related to Christ Consciousness.

✤ Pentagonal Dodecahedron (twelve pentagonal faces)—also contains the parameters of the DNA and represents ether and the female. This shape is also related to Christ Consciousness.

If you were to add a sphere to this list, it would represent the void and child aspect of nature. This is all written in detailed description in the book *The Ancient Secret of the Flower of Life*. You can also do a simple Internet search to understand the broader connection between geometry and the origins of the Universe. Here, I just want you to have a basic understanding of how sacred geometry is part of the production of your baby and is linked to the emotional, physical, mental and spiritual aspects of creation. Each shape has a relationship to who you are. In this book, we break down this complex geometry to its simplest forms in order to connect it back to yourself. My intention is to make you lighter and a walking representation of nature in balance. My hope is that you become a happier individual and a better mother. We will use alchemy to return you to your truest self.

Creating the Crystalline Child

Awakened human beings have a sensitive sensory system that allows a higher level of creativity and knowing to flow through them. These individuals often create genius inventions for humanity in the fields of art or science. Einstein and Tesla could not have birthed new and brilliant ideas into the world without having the magnetic auric architecture that could hold and place these concepts into form. They required a connection to something larger than themselves to allow this inspiration to flow through.

Reflect on Michelangelo creating the Sistine Chapel. In order for him to complete this, he would have had to see the art in his mind's eye long before he painted it. He would have also had to experience these heavenly realms in a fifth-dimensional and palpable way to create something so magnificent. This would have required him to taste the experience in his mouth, feel that intense desire in his body and hear the sounds of choirs of angels singing. All of these sensations were required to design, or birth, something that had never been conceived on Earth before. The Sistine Chapel was Michelangelo's baby.

In order for you to create a human unlike any other, you need to begin to imagine this child now and fully engage your sensory system in the creation process. You can ask for the exact type of child you would like to conceive and create. Even if you are currently pregnant, you can still do this because the soul of the child does not enter the body until the 120th day after conception according to yogic philosophy (I discuss this in *Mystical Motherhood* in detail). After this point in time, meditation, mantras (or sacred sounds), positive thoughts and prayer during pregnancy can help to clear the karma of your child and amplify his or her destiny before birth.

Think of someone in history who has created something absolutely brilliant— perhaps a writer, a singer or a poet. Imagine your very favorite book or piece of art. When this artist was painting, cooking or playing music, what type of sensory experience were they having? It was likely highly engaged and connected to Spirit. The reason that you love their creations or masterpieces is because you can feel the same connection they had when you experience the art in the present moment. This is timelessness, this is God, and this is what I would like you to emulate before conception and during pregnancy.

Let's compare creating an enlightened child to writing a piece of music like Mozart or Alicia Keys. Alicia cannot create something that is long-lasting unless her energy is running at a high vibration. In order to create music that others will respond to, she has to literally hear, taste, see, feel, and touch these sounds. She has to be fully awake, in her divine mind, and connected to her Higher Self. She also has to feel how others will respond to this movement in motion in all space and time. Her music is her baby and the vibration she is running at the time of creating this child is the result of her work. When extraordinary people connect Heaven on Earth the Holy Trinity is born.

You will not be able to create a piece of art, or an enlightened child, if your vibration is not running at a high speed at the time of conception or pregnancy. All of the best inventions or pieces of art carry the frequency of their creator. It takes discipline and inspiration to birth a masterpiece. The greatest artists on Earth strive for perfection. From this point forward, you must work to enhance your sensory system. This is an important part of raising your vibration in order to attract a higher vibrational child.

The Visualization to Create an Enlightened Child detailed earlier should have provided you with an initial baseline of your frequency which would indicate the type of child you would currently attract and create. At the end of this section, I will ask you to review your life and the types of sensations that the people, places, and things you surround yourself with create within your body. This is important to pay attention to because, as you will soon learn, your surrounding environment affects your DNA. Ensuring that the people you spend your time with are kind and your physical environment is calm is very important before and during pregnancy because your thoughts, emotions and beliefs program your baby. It is important for you to improve some areas in your life, such as your work and home environment and relationship to self and others, because they will ultimately affect the vibration of the child inside of you.

Understanding Your Frequency or Vibration

Before we move on to assessing and improving your environment and senses, however, I want to briefly define what vibration is—as I comprehend it and as it was described to me in an interview with Dr. Celestine Star[3]. Your vibration may be invisible, but it affects everything and everyone, just as other people's vibrations affect you. There are five archetypes of creation, or vibrations, that design your specific frequency. Understanding these will provide you with a better visual of your energy. You will also be able to determine why you would attract a high-caliber soul and if you would actually be able to hold this soul's energy within your body without suffering from a pregnancy loss. I am not indicating here that all miscarriages are a result of an energetic mismatch between mother and baby—I am just pointing out that this is a possibility.

Everything in our world is made up of a waveform or pattern that has a certain signature or sound. Reality as a whole is just different wavelengths. As you go up through dimensions, the wavelengths become shorter with higher energy. As

---

3   (Star, 2018)

you go down in the dimensions the wavelengths get longer with lower energy. The various dimensional levels have to do with harmonics or music. Earth is in the third dimension and has a denser waveform and frequency. Think of objects such as a book, body or couch, which are made up of tiny atoms. These physical objects make up planet Earth as we know it. Those in higher dimensions do not experience this density in the same manner. The five archetypes of creation that make up these waveforms of energy include: electric, magnetic, radial, wave, and steady[4]. Getting the right frequency will help you become pregnant and attract a high-caliber soul from higher dimensions.

The Five Archetypes of Creation

ELECTRIC: This type of frequency looks like fire. In your mind's eye, imagine that you are outside sitting around a camp fire staring at the flames. You may begin to notice that the fire actually contains many colors within it. It is blue or green at the bottom and radiates outward into orange and red. The bottom of the flames have a shorter wave pattern and are more solid in nature. As this electric energy moves out in its unidirectional form, it becomes higher in vibration and looser towards the ends. You can visualize this now by imagining the tips of each of the flames as they rapidly move towards the top of the fire. When you are trying to conceive, you want to have a solid electric current of energy that has a shorter wave pattern. In other words, you want to hold the type of energy that is similar to the blue at the bottom of the fire rather than the erratic movement of the bright red that is found at the tips of fire. A solid electrical current is more stable.

I asked various women to complete *The Visualization to Create an Enlightened Child*, in order to determine the type of soul they would attract at the moment of conception. Everyone's experience was completely different. A few said that they saw a red and electric energy entering the room. This signified to me that their current frequency is not stable, which may make it hard to actually hold a child in the womb. The women who experienced this red electric current also had an

---

4 (Star, 2018)

unstable life with a flighty and fast disposition, often jumping from one career or relationship to the next. They tended to be very anxious and emotionally unpredictable. To conceive and hold a high-frequency child, it is better to have a solid vibrational field, which is evident in a grounded and centered woman.

MAGNETIC: This is dense energy that is connected to love and the center of creation. It creates a container and is the cause of gravity. If you demagnetize yourself, you will literally begin floating. In other words, if you were to change your waveform of consciousness and alter your body pattern to match that of a higher dimensional field, you could disappear out of the third dimension and arrive in the one that you tuned into.

If you have a magnetic energy, things will come to you easily. Life will flow in your favor because you are not energetically inclined to repel opportunities. If you find that nothing goes your way, you may need to work on your frequency. Individuals who are magnetic find themselves in the right place and the right time. Magnetism has the potential to create miracles because of the amount of opportunity and luck that is attracted.

Magnetism creates protection through its circular and attractive energy, which literally becomes a point at which all things meet or are created. An actual physical example of magnetism is a house—a magnetic wavelength that is a solid structure and protective in nature. You want your womb to be a powerful magnetic container and the tissue should exemplify this energy.

RADIAL: This is circular radial energy always going outwards—similar to the way that circular motions occur on the water of a pool or lake. The tones of radial waves create sound patterns that extend out like the flower of life. When you are pregnant, you are creating the hologram of the child within you. During this period, much of your energy goes to the center of your womb allowing the cells to communicate and come together as the creation of your child perfectly unfolds. A balanced energy field is important, especially before conception. If your energy is being directed only from your head, throat, or solar plexus, it could be harder to become pregnant or have a balanced pregnancy.

Sine wave: This is a feminine energy that carries information or a codex. Sine waves move from one radial point outwards and correspond to light or the electromagnetic spectrum. Everything in creation is a sine wave. The only thing that makes one sine wave differ from another is its pattern. These differentiations create cell communication. This is how mental projections from the brain occur, fingers move, and organs function—the entire body is created via geometrical construction in your womb.

Steady: This is God energy and is not destructible. It is the magnetic idea that birthed you into the world. When you become your God-Self you produce that God-Self within your womb. If your energy is steady like the ethereal realms, you are going to create God Consciousness within you.

To sum up everything I have discussed thus far, I want to make the following clear: 1) The base frequency and characteristics of your child are created at conception and within the first few days of creation. 2) The soul you attract is based on your energetic signature. 3) You can continue to clear the soul you are carrying of his or her karma, and everything that you would pass down to the baby, while you are pregnant. This is done through a strong spiritual practice and the recommendations put forth in this book and *Mystical Motherhood*. 4) The more preparation that you do before you become pregnant the better. I believe that the release of mental, emotional, physical and spiritual density will increase your fertility.

Exercise: Questions to Enhance the Six Senses

Your surroundings affect your senses, and optimizing your physical environment will raise the vibration of your emotional, mental, and spiritual bodies. You will learn later in the book how your environment programs your DNA. An awakened individual has a heightened sensory system, which creates intuition and a connection to higher dimensions. There are six sides to the cube that is a representation of the physical body, and there are six senses. These senses provide your body with its unique ability to interact with earth and your surroundings. They provide a platform for the physical body here on Earth. In their purest form, the senses can function at highly acute levels. This is what makes people clairvoyant or clairaudient. This is also partially the reason that some individuals are excellent artists, singers, cooks or builders. They have a heightened awareness in their specific fields. Answer the following questions in your journal and begin to think of ways that you can heighten your senses or improve your environment.

Vision

· What are you looking at all day? Is it a computer screen or desk?

· Do you spend any time in meditation engaging your third eye—the space between your eyebrows—so that you can really begin to see the unseen through meditation?

· What type of area do you live in (city or countryside)? Are your home, work, and surroundings nice to be in or look at?

· Describe your current home and how it affects your senses.

· How can you improve these areas of your life? Perhaps you could surround yourself with more physical beauty?

Hearing or Sound

· What types of music do you listen to and what are the general sounds in your environment? Do you pay attention to the sounds of the birds or are you too preoccupied?

· Who do you spend your time talking to and what types of words come out of your mouth or theirs?

· Do you speak negatively about others or are you careful—only saying and listening to positive uplifting words or sounds? Make a note of the types of conversations you have had with friends or family over the past month. Were the words you used uplifting? How can you improve this?

· In general, what do you do in your spare time? If you had the option, would you go to a loud bar on a Saturday afternoon or would you go on a hike? How often do you choose a better physical environment and how does this affect your senses?

Taste

· What types of foods are you commonly eating? Keep a general list of what your taste buds currently enjoy. How does this connect to your overall demeanor? Do you tend to be sour, reactive, harsh or critical?

· Do you feel weighed down by the density of your diet? Do you pick intoxicants that numb your system such as drugs or alcohol?

· Could you improve the vibrational quality of your food and the types of products you allow into your body?

Smell and Touch

· Do you pay attention to your environment and the smells around you? How can you enhance this?

· What types of items do you keep around the house? What are the textures of your clothes and bedding?

· Is your office or place of work filled with beautiful items? How could you improve this: perhaps with flowers?

Proprioception

· Where is your body in space and time and what is your awareness of your surroundings? How are you moving through your environment? Are your movements subtle or pronounced?

· What is your body in relationship to the matrix—the world around you? If you think of yourself as a hologram, your body is the level of density that you hold in this holographic field. It is also the relationship you have to the objects around you and space in general. It is what holds you down to earth. How physically dense is your body?

Exercise: Paint a Canvas of your Child

You have the ability to attract a specific type of soul down to the planet. I would like you to begin to fully sense the type of child that you would like to conceive and create. What does this child feel like to you as you use all of your senses?

Many of the clients I work with that are struggling with fertility, or who have lost children in miscarriages, are afraid of imagining their child because they cannot handle the loss of their dream. Manifestation requires feeling, sensing and seeing something before it happens. Your thoughts create your Reality. This is also true for having a child. Create your child by projecting from the level of your heart—not your head. Manifesting from your head brings polarity and you will always create the opposite of what you want. When you create or speak your desires from your heart, they become real and are pure without the polarization.

In your mind's eye project a circle from the level of your heart with a high energetic frequency. Watch as it turns into a vesica piscis and cells divide into a cube and continually create a vast amount of sacred geometrical shapes which become the fetus of your child. Watch your child grow in your mind's eye and place this baby into your womb. Fill your baby with the type of energy you wish to hold. If you would like to bring down a scientist, painter, healer or leader you can ask for this. You can also ask for the child to bring health, wealth, and happiness to your family.

CHAPTER 2

SCIENCE

Behavioral Epigenetics: The Emerging Scientific Field

According to Bruce Lipton, author of *The Biology of Belief*, a cell's life is controlled by its physical and energetic environment with only a small portion managed by its genes. He discovered this while working with cells in petri dishes. When he created a healthy environment for cells, they thrived. When he did not, they struggled. By readjusting the conditions for the cells in his petri dishes, he could make sick cells well again. This ultimately means that cells are responsive and change according to their environmental signals. Understanding this is critical before you become pregnant, because it means that the cells within your growing fetus, which are quadrupling at a massive rate every second, can be programmed. This is something that the ancient yogis have always known, but now science is catching up. Environmental signals that affect cells are thoughts, beliefs, emotions, and nutrition, because all of these things are a form of energy. Bruce Lipton's discovery was a game changer because it marked the beginning of the merging of the fields of science and Spirit.

His work, called behavioral epigenetics, has become one of the fastest growing areas of scientific research. This field is showing that genes are dynamic and responsive to everything that you think and do. Epigenetics demonstrates that you are in control of your gene activity and can enhance your genome through a better connection to your body, mind, and spirit. You must begin to think of these three attributes of Self as parts of one system as they are constantly interacting and communicating, similar to a computer or telephone network. Everything you eat, think or feel is received by this system, creating messages and memories that are being sent directly to your DNA. Our genome holds the memories of our ancestors and most often, we pass these memories on to our children. In this book, I will show you various ways that you can heal yourself and clear these memories from your epigenetic line before you have your next child.

I grew up with the belief system that because my grandma had heart disease I could easily inherit it. I also had a fear that I would automatically inherit or experience the diabetes, mental illness, and high cholesterol that run in my genetic line. According to this new research, that is not the case. Behavioral epigenetics is proving that DNA works more like a light switch that can be turned on or off. There are a few inheritable diseases that will automatically be passed down from one generation to the next, but the vast amount of your personality and health attributes are malleable. A genetic variant in your DNA strand can predispose you to certain diseases or behaviors, but it doesn't mean that you are guaranteed to have these issues in your life. Your personal DNA is like a blueprint, giving a small percentage of fixed characteristics, such as brown eyes or blonde hair.

If you are considering ordering a genetic test to understand your DNA, you should know the following: doctors are only able to provide the *probability* that you will develop a disease when looking over your genetic constitution. The presence of the BRCA1 gene, which is the gene for breast cancer, doesn't mean that the person will necessarily develop the disease[5]. It indicates that the segment is faulty and the person has an increased risk. DNA cannot single-handedly cause disease. Genetic material does not predict what will happen: it is the context of your life as a whole that will determine whether a specific gene will turn on or off.

We are affected by the awareness we have of our environment, our perception of what is happening around us, and our responses to environmental signals[6]. Transferring this knowledge to pregnancy means that if you improve the environment for the fetus, you can ultimately change the DNA. Our cells change in

---

5   (Moore, 2015)

6   (Lipton, 2015)

response to our experiences, which should begin to give you a better understanding of why each of us develops the unique characteristics that we do.

The New School

I was not taught this emerging field of science in my undergraduate biology class. Behavioral epigenetics was not even mentioned more recently as I studied for my Master's in Nursing or my Family Nurse Practitioner degree. I guarantee this is not what medical students are now learning in school either. This is truly disappointing, because the implications are mind boggling. We can no longer give ourselves excuses for not living to our full potential. Lipton explains that we are not frail individuals being passed defective genes from previous generations. We are actually powerful creators of our own reality and have the potential to turn genes off and on for higher functioning. Your physical, emotional, and spiritual well-being can actually determine whether or not diseases will be expressed in your health. While you contemplate that you have this kind of power over the expression of your genes, I also want you to begin to consider the effect you can have on the environment of your growing child while he or she is still inside you.

In order to understand where we are today, and how fast science has changed, we must understand our history and where the theory that genes control our future came from. It goes back to the 1800s when *The Origin of Species* was published. Darwin stated that individual traits are passed from parents to their children. These hereditary factors were deemed to control existence and this became the central belief system of biology[7]. Darwin believed that it would take many generations for genes to shift. What epigenetics is proving is that it can happen in just one generation. You have the power to change the generational patterns for your children in this lifetime.

There has always been a debate between nature vs. nurture, but for a scientist holding fast in the belief that destiny is in the hands of DNA, nature usually won. As a society, we have been programmed to believe that one day genes will turn on us and we will inherit what our father had, or give our children what we were

---

7   (Moore, 2015)

diagnosed with. There are a few specific diseases that are a result of genetics. However, the cause of most diseases is actually the relationship among multiple genes and their environment. Only five percent of cancer and cardiovascular patients can attribute their disease to genetics. Ninety-five percent of breast cancers are not due to inherited genes[8]. Simply by changing our diet and lifestyle, we can avoid serious illness. Epigenetics is demonstrating that we can alter DNA through thoughts, emotions, environment and food. In this book, you will learn how to apply this to your pregnancy.

The Human Genome Project was a global scientific effort started in the 1980s that aimed to catalogue all the genes within a human. Scientists thought that the genome would contain one hundred and twenty thousand genes located within two pairs of twenty-three chromosomes. They were shocked when they found that the entire genome of a human consists of fewer than twenty-five thousand genes. This meant that eighty percent of the DNA they thought was required for humans does not exist[9]. Scientists discovered that we are genetically similar to primitive organisms and that our DNA can be compared to that of rodents, as both species have a similar number of genes. This obviously shocked the scientific community. A grain of rice has more than double the number of genes than a human[10]. The evolution of the human DNA has become efficient at gene expression and allows us to biologically function at a higher rate with comparatively fewer genes than other creations on this planet. What we once understood about our existence is changing and it is happening very fast.

Basic Information on the Functions of DNA

We need evolution on this planet and we cannot have this without gene mutation. Our ancestors developed insulin resistance in order to survive famines. A mutation in the genes was required for basic survival. Now this mutation is causing some of us not to be able to zip up our pants. Was this mutation a good thing

---

8   (Moore, 2015)

9   (Moore, 2015)

10   (Tanzi, 2015)

or a bad thing? We know that our genes will adapt to their environment and we can choose to create super humans or see what happens over time as our bodies continuously take on the environmental toxins that are increasing at great speed.

Epigenetics controls your genes, makes you incredibly unique, and is a reversible process. I am going to teach you a few simple things about the biology of cells so you have a basic understanding of how DNA works on a micro level. If this doesn't interest you, skip this section. It is not my goal to get you bored—just very informed as to what you will be scientifically activating within the cells when you apply this book to your everyday life. There are rows of books in libraries written on the following; I have attempted to break it down for you to make it as accessible as possible. You must understand that there are no good genes or bad genes—it is just the mutation in the DNA sequence or structure that can cause some good genes to go bad.

How our Environment Affects DNA

It was once thought that the flow of information within cells was unidirectional, but now science is finding that a cell's DNA, RNA and proteins function in a completely different manner. According to David Moore, author of *The Developing Genome*, the new model is more sophisticated: alteration to the DNA strand starts with an environmental signal, which goes to a regulatory protein which changes the DNA, RNA, and the resulting protein. Scientists were missing the first two steps of gene alteration before this finding. They had not realized that the environmental signal was critical to altering DNA strands.

Understanding the microbiological role of regulatory proteins is important because they can create two thousand or more variations of proteins from the exact same blueprint of genes. This means that your DNA code maintains the exact same blueprint your whole life, but can be expressed, transmitted or modified in many ways depending on your environmental input[11]. Approximately ninety-nine percent of human DNA is exactly the same from person to person. Approximately one percent is different.

---

11   (Moore, 2015)

This small percentage creates the variances in our DNA and makes each person unique. Variants in DNA are what make the subtle differences within populations. Some variants in the DNA will predispose you to certain health problems, others will do nothing at all. The expression of these variances within DNA is generally activated by what we do, how we experience the world, and our environmental exposures. It is difficult to predict how genes will actually express themselves within a person because it is this combination, plus the interaction with many genes on a microscopic scale that create these variants or mutations.

The Regulation of Gene Expression

The methylation of DNA affects how genes are expressed or not. It is a mechanism used by cells to control gene expression. There are different epigenetic mechanisms that can activate or inactivate DNA. When a methyl group attaches to a gene segment, it essentially "silences" it or inactivates it most of the time. On the other hand, when histones, or proteins, within the DNA chain are methylated, they cause increased gene activation. This process ultimately, then, turns genes off or on. This can be good or bad for your health, depending on what gene is being manipulated.

A team of researchers in Madrid published a report on the epigenetic statuses of forty pairs of identical twins. These twins were born with identical sets of genes, which we once thought would predestine them to be exactly the same the rest of their lives. Findings show that this is not the case. When the twins were young, they had similar DNA strands, but as they grew older, the epigenetic markings gradually became markedly different as a result of living different lifestyles[12]. This is because each twin had a different experience of the world, which then affected the expression of their genes. This study demonstrates that experiences leave marks on our DNA, which affect how our genes are expressed.

---

12   (Moore, 2015)

DNA Replication

An individual's experiences also affect their telomeres, which are structures at the end of chromosomes. They do not code and are called "junk" DNA. Telomeres are important because they prevent the DNA from unwinding and provide the platform for DNA to replicate. In order for a gene to reproduce itself, it must make duplicate DNA strands to ensure that each daughter cell receives the complete genome. Each time the DNA strand is copied, it becomes shorter, which could make the cell become dysfunctional. When this was discovered, scientists thought that our life spans should not be very long, but this was before they found the unique function of an enzyme in our body named telomerase[13]. This powerful enzyme helps to extend the length of telomeres. Telomerase replenishes telomeres and increases vitality within the cell. It can ultimately enhance health and extend life.

Bruce Lipton explained this further when he said, "Life experiences can stimulate or suppress telomerase activity. For example, stressful prenatal developmental experiences, childhood abuse (both verbal and physical), domestic violence, post-traumatic stress disorder (PTSD), nutritional deficiencies and lack of love all inhibit telomerase activity. These factors contribute to the onset of disease and a shortened life span. In contrast, exercise, good nutrition, a positive outlook on life, living in happiness and gratitude, being in service, and experiencing love, especially self-love, all enhance telomerase activity and promote a long and healthy life." Our environment matters to even the enzyme telomerase: that is how powerful our perception is.

Science is proving on a microscopic level that our cells are affected by their environment. In a study done at Duke University, scientists studied the DNA of a group of children at age five and then at age ten, knowing that some of these children experienced abuse, bullying or violent domestic disputes. They found that the children who had had these stressful life experiences had reduced and eroded telomere length[14]. Other research has shown that meditation and exercise

---

13   (Lipton, 2015)

14   (Tanzi & Chopra, 2015)

can increase the length of telomeres. Life experiences have a profound effect on our bodies at the most microscopic levels and the implications of these findings are important for you to understand as a parent.

Applying Behavioral Epigenetics to Pregnancy

Bruce Lipton demonstrated in his research that cells are primarily molded by their environment, not by the DNA that is held within them. I have just described how this works scientifically, and now I will apply the concepts you have learned regarding behavioral epigenetics to the growth period of pregnancy. You can affect the child in your womb during pregnancy by improving your internal (thoughts, emotions and beliefs) and external (food and toxins) environmental inputs. I believe that the environment of your growing child will also be affected by your sensory awareness. Amplifying your awareness of taste, touch and surrounding sounds, sights and smells before and during pregnancy could ultimately create environmental inputs that could program your child with heightened awareness of the senses and perception of his or her environment later in life.

In our mother's womb, we all begin life as a fertilized egg, which is a cell. Within the nucleus of this cell are the chromosomes contributed by our parents. This egg develops into an adult that is made up of trillions of cells. Within every one of those cells is the same set of genes from the original cell[15]. In the Spirit section of the book you learned that the consciousness of these original eight cells is critical to creating enlightened children. You can energetically affect this universal series of events, and enhance the awareness of your cells, by reducing the physical, emotional, mental and spiritual density that you hold within your body. The consciousness of your cells will ultimately create the consciousness of your child's, because as you now know cells adjust and change according to their surroundings. You have the ability to optimize your body, mind, and spirit before conception and during pregnancy in order to create the healthiest child with a stronger genome.

---

15   (Moore, 2015)

Lipton compared the cell to a computer because both are programmed by a source from outside themselves. You can think of each cell in your body as a computer chip. Data can be edited at any point. During pregnancy, the fetus grows at an astonishing rate, replicating cells every second. The brain of a baby in utero grows at the rate of two-hundred and fifty-thousand nerve cells per minute. This is by far the most critical time of human development. Applying these astonishing, and relatively new, scientific findings should be of the utmost importance to you.

The time between conception and birth creates the characteristics and destiny of the child for a lifetime. The spiritual and energetic work that you do before and during pregnancy will give your child a head-start in life. He or she will be far ahead of other adults who are held back by the density they carry within them from previous generations. The ancient yogis and holy communities throughout history knew this. Women who wanted to bring advanced souls to Earth would spend a significant amount of time in meditation or prayer. You can learn more about all of this by visiting the Mystical Motherhood website, where there is a vast amount of audio, visual, and reading material dedicated to ancient yogic science and creating an enhanced human being.

Pregnancy is the most crucial period of development and possibly the missing link to creating an enhanced individual—and even an enhanced world population. Sadly, the importance of this time period is not the focus of the current Western medical system. My intention is that this book will change that. While I was in nursing school and training to become a Family Nurse Practitioner, I never once heard a professor teach that the thoughts, emotions, or stress level of the pregnant mother matter. Western medical professionals care about whether the patient is meeting testing parameters and statistics. They follow a basic protocol for prenatal visits. Depending on what phase of pregnancy you are in, you will receive a series of tests to determine the fetus's level of health and well-being. The medical community is missing what is happening on an emotional, mental, and spiritual level to the mother and her baby. This can't be quantified; thus it will not be tested.

Medical professionals typically do not ask about the working conditions, home environment or internal stressors of the pregnant mother. If a woman was in fact in danger, scared or stressed during pregnancy, she would likely be passed on to another medical professional who might or might not be able to get her out of that situation. There are too many cracks in our system and many people fall between. It is up to you to create the ultimate health for your family. Most doctors will not approach new ideas that have not been scientifically proven and tested. The problem with the information I have discussed is that it is subjective: each person's personal awareness differs vastly from another's, and as a result it is difficult to quantify scientifically.

Despite what society and the medical community believe, motherhood does not start at birth—it begins at conception. Cells are responsive and conscious, so everything you think and feel will literally be creating the type of child you will birth into this world. Would you allow your toddler to be around a physical fight or watch a violent movie? Would you tell your child that they look fat, that you don't like them, or you hate their existence? If you think these types of negative thoughts towards yourself or others, or if you place yourself in these violent environments during pregnancy, you are not being the most aware mother. You are naturally going to program or affect the cells of your growing child in utero, and it is up to you whether you are conscious about the data you put in or not.

Negative thoughts, emotions and diet are hard to change overnight. You cannot assume that when you become pregnant you will automatically become a better person. It takes a significant amount of time and discipline to improve your lifestyle and environmental input. Women spend most of their pregnancy preparing for the birth of their child and the transition into becoming a parent. I want to flip this paradigm and have you begin to prepare for motherhood long before conception by changing your entire approach to health and personal well-being. If you are already pregnant, it is not too late to start. You are now in Parenting Class 101 and school is in session. This is your modern guide to conscious motherhood.

BODY — THE SQUARE

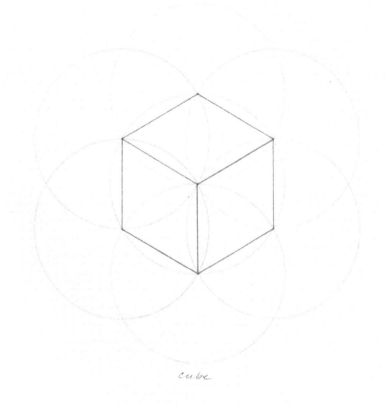

cube

CHAPTER 3

NUTRITION

Food's Epigenetic Effects on Anatomy and Behavior

It is vital to discuss your nutritional state before conception and during pregnancy when it comes to the health and well-being of yourself and your child. The quantity of what you are eating may or may not be meeting your body's requirements. The quality of your food can help you to reach higher spiritual states of consciousness. A key factor to raising your vibration and reducing your physical density comes down to what you eat and drink. Nutrition, especially an anti-inflammatory diet, will create internal clarity, and cleaning up your diet and reducing toxins will help you to conceive consciously.

If you are having trouble becoming pregnant, balancing your weight and nutrient levels should be your priority. If you are already pregnant, nutrition is not often spoken about in detail during prenatal visits. I hope to include enough information here so that you can make some valuable changes in a stepwise approach that doesn't feel overwhelming. Understanding what to eat and what to avoid will not only help to enhance your gut microbiome, levels of happiness and frequency, but also your DNA.

Food has epigenetic effects on your genome and there is a vast amount of research to prove it. In 2003, a study done on rodents demonstrated how diet can alter the expression of mutant genes. A group of mice were born with yellow fur, and a very large appetite that made them obese. These rodents were fed standard mouse food, but one group was given nutritional methyl supplements including vitamin B12, choline and folic acid. The offspring of the mice that had been given the supplements grew to have brown fur and normal weight. The mother's nutritional state had a profound impact on her children's health. This study demonstrated how each generation contributes genetically to the next. The rodents given supplements experienced epigenetic changes, radically different-looking appearances and health improvements compared to the control group. The methyl supplement in this study silenced or modified the DNA, reducing the incidence of diabetes, obesity, and cancer in the rodents[16].

Honeybees are a particularly interesting example of the effects of epigenetics on anatomy and behavior. All of the bees within a hive are identical—clones of one another. A small number of the bees become queen bees who do not look the same as, and behave differently from, their sister worker bees. This is because the queens consume a different diet called royal jelly, full of a specific protein. As a result, they have larger abdomens, a lifespan that is twenty times longer, and mature ovaries that can reproduce. The worker bees have a shorter lifespan, produce stingers and pollen baskets. The protein in the jelly causes demethylation on specific genes in the queens, altering their expression, and making these genetically identical bees different from their sister worker bees[17]. It is not the diet alone that accounts for this difference, but the interaction of this diet with the genome of the bees.

There is research that shows the effect of food on the human genome too. During World War II, the Dutch faced drastic food shortages and famine as supplies to the area stopped. Scientists studied the children of the Dutch famine showing that DNA changes that happen in an adult's life can be inherited by the next generation. The health records showed that babies born at that time suffered from severe health problems. The children were born larger and heavier than average and as they grew into adults they were highly prone to obesity[18]. These effects were more profound in individuals who were in the womb spe-

---

16   (Tanzi, 2015)

17   (Moore, 2015)

18   (Tanzi, 2015)

cifically in the second and third trimester, compared to the first. The prenatal experiences of these individuals programmed them to experience scarcity in the form of nutrition.

The Consequences of an Unhealthy Diet

Poor in-utero nutrition can contribute to childhood obesity. This applies to both women who do not eat enough and those who consistently make unhealthy choices, such as junk food. In both cases the babies experience nutrient deficiencies. Children born to overweight mothers are epigenetically programmed to build adipose tissue at birth. When the mother is not getting enough of the right nutrients for health, the child inside feels the scarcity. He or she will always be feeling this on a cellular level and may consistently be desiring food later in life. (This is just a theory, but it wouldn't surprise me if this programmed scarcity is also transferred to other emotional desires manifesting in relationships and material items). The mother actually programs the child to be overweight because in utero the baby never had enough.

Many of the women who eat fast food in pregnancy could actually be significantly harming their children. Research has shown a high level of endotoxin, a word that means inner poison, in individuals after eating at McDonald's[19]. When endotoxin is found in the body, the immune system immediately believes that a foreign invader has arrived. This results in a significant amount of inflammation within the body. Inflammation in turn negatively affects the microbiome and thus the DNA of the cells, creating health consequences. One in four Americans eats fast food regularly. If you do, reducing this high carbohydrate, sugar, and trans-fat diet during pregnancy could be as critical to your health during this period as stopping the consumption of alcohol or drugs.

---

19   (M.D. C. S., 2008)

Nutrient Depletion in Pregnancy

Approximately seventy-four percent of American women are lacking proper nutrients in their diet. The effects of this level of depletion may not be apparent in your current state of health, but at some moment in time down the genetic chain someone in your family will suffer from this level of loss. Our genome has been maltreated for too many years, which may be the cause of the massive reproduction issues we are now experiencing. Each generation will suffer more if we don't start to pay closer attention to our body's needs. It is only natural that we will start to see more problems with health in years to come, as individuals will likely begin to physically age faster, suffer emotionally and develop diseases at higher rates. In order to protect your children, you not only need to eat right, but you also must consider spacing your children or fully replenishing your nutrient levels between each pregnancy.

In the Western culture, it is common for women to have babies later in life. As a result of this, if they choose to have multiple children, they are birthing them closer together. This does not allow for their bodies to build up proper nutrient reserves, which affects the child's genome and the mother's health. Catherine Shanahan explained in her book *Deep Nutrition: Why Your Genes Need Nutritional Food* that the fetus behaves similarly to a parasite within the womb—oblivious to the health of the host. The baby will take whatever it needs in order to survive. Each pregnancy drains the mother's body of vital vitamins and minerals unless she takes the time and energy to replenish.

You will possibly have enough nutrients for your first baby, but will likely be depleted after having more children if you don't renew your level of health. The women of some tribal cultures naturally understood this. They made efforts to separate the births of their children by three to four years in order to ensure that their bodies would have enough time to nutritionally build themselves back up. They did this to protect the health of their future generations and their genome. If a diet is deficient in fat, the fetus will extract fat as needed from the mother's brain. If the baby needs calcium he or she will take the nutrients from the mother's bones if necessary.

The placenta was created to protect the child and has supernatural nutrient scavenging abilities. Even in an environment with poor nutrition, the first child will likely thrive. It's the following offspring that will experience the disadvantage, especially if the woman's storehouse of nutrients was not refilled. If there are not enough nutrients, the second child's epigenetic expression will likely be impaired, which may cause disease or disability throughout his or her life. Shanahan explained that the subsequent children of a woman lacking a proper nutrient storehouse will be constructed as best as possible under the conditions; however, both the mother and the child may suffer as a result. We have no idea what will happen to the future generations if we do not learn to eat a diet that is nutrient rich like our ancestors.

Shanahan discussed the importance of creating a birth gap between pregnancies in order to restore the nutrient levels of the mother's body for each child and her own well-being. She said, "Previous studies have shown that births less than eighteen months apart increase child mortality and, in some cases, stunt growth." She noted facial disproportions, variances in appearance and skeletal structural asymmetry in second- and third-born children. These subtle symmetry shifts can cause injury or pain later in life. The underlying cause of these structural problems is not because of the birth order, but a result of malnourishment of the mother which affects the child in the womb. Systematic spacing of children and planning are forms of female empowerment and freedom.

What Doctors Have Not Told You

Sadly, nutrition is not a big focus in Western medical school for nurses or doctors. In fact, as far as I remember, it was just a basic prerequisite and the subject was rarely mentioned in school or within the clinic. In order for Western medical practitioners to understand all the facets of nutrition, they have to do their own research, but with so many patients to see and such little time, this becomes difficult. It seems that most individuals only begin to care about nutrition when they start to get sick. When this happens, because of lack of time with patients, medical professionals hand out pills, when the root cause of the problem could likely be healed through some internal stress management and a better diet.

I was working with a client who had not had her menstrual cycle for over a year, suffered from stomach pain, and experienced fear of food for almost two years. We will call her Sara. Sara had been to many professionals in the hopes of becoming pregnant, but no one asked her about her diet. She started working with me because she was desperately ready to have a baby. At our first session, on the phone, I energetically scanned her and saw immediately that her cells needed nutrition. I explained that she needed to gain weight as her body mass index was way too low. Sara said that no one else had mentioned this. Her fear of food and need to control what she ate, stemmed from her childhood and her relationship with her mother. When she recognized that her mother's need to control was a part of her current fears around food she began to heal. She also understood just how depleted her body was after having her first baby, breastfeeding and losing weight because of an illness. Her realizations and path of internal healing helped her to gain over twenty pounds, which balanced her hormones and brought back her menstrual cycle.

It is concerning to me that most practitioners lead their pregnant patients to believe that a prenatal vitamin is going to be enough to protect their health. It is not. It is also upsetting that we don't encourage women to boost their nutrient level or clean up their diet before each pregnancy. Since most practitioners are not going to ask you about your diet, or help you make necessary changes, it is up to you to protect your own health and that of your future generations. The best way to create optimal health is to eat whole foods that do not cause inflammation. Since most of us didn't grow up learning what this means, I am going to do my very best to explain as much as I can here. I will list what you should and should not eat to prepare your body for pregnancy and amplify your DNA to create ultimate health. The breadth of this book cannot include all the information required, so I encourage you to read the references I have provided.

The Connection Between Your Microbiome and DNA

Your body is made up of almost one hundred trillion cells and many of these are found in the lining of your gut and on the surface of your skin. For optimal health, these cells need to function properly, and if they are constantly attacked by toxins that cause inflammation, they cannot. The bacteria in your gut is also known as microbiome which assists with digestion and is key to your health. In order for cells to properly function, they look to your body's DNA, most of which is tucked inside of the bacteria in your microbiome.

Deepak Chopra explained in his book *Super Genes*, "It is estimated that ninety percent of the genetic information found inside is bacterial—our ancestors were microbes, and they are still present in the sculpture of our cells." You can protect your gut bacteria with a diet that is high in healthy fats and plant-based foods. By improving your diet, you will improve or maintain a strong genome because much of your DNA is held within the cells or bacteria of your gut. You have twenty-three thousand genes inside your cells and one million genes for the vast number of microbes found in your digestive system[20].

Food is a language. It is a powerful code that programs your cells. You have the ability to upgrade your system and protect your genome by eating the right diet. If you were to eliminate anti-inflammatory foods, or even just switch to a primarily vegetarian-based diet, you would see an improvement in the health of your microbiome in just days. We are no longer eating the way our ancestors did, and the high amount of toxins and lack of minerals are going to drastically affect coming generations. The foods that we are currently eating are depleted in nutrients and sourced from some very questionable places.

DO YOU EAT ANY OF THE FOLLOWING?

* Frozen, canned or vitamin-poor fruits and vegetables

* Mystery meats packaged from farms with poisoned animals

* Grains grown in mineral-depleted soils

* Soy products

* Packaged goods (breakfast cereal, chips, granola or crackers)

* Artificially flavored candies or snacks

---

20   (Tanzi, 2015)

- ✤ Fat-free anything and everything

- ✤ Margarine

- ✤ French fries anyone?

- ✤ White bread or white rice

- ✤ Monosodium glutamate (MSG)

If you do, you may still be alright because your grandparents likely ate well enough to maintain your genome. No one can guarantee that your future generations will be able to handle the nutrient deficiencies or toxins much longer though. If you have not experienced any problems yet, consider yourself lucky. Perhaps you know someone who has suffered? Do your family members or friends have any health problems or perhaps their children? There has been a rise in birth defects, asthma, autism, childhood depression, obesity, heart disease, diabetes, and allergies[21]. You must know someone with a child who is suffering from an ailment that could likely be changed through food. I know I do.

Reduce Your Inflammation

It is impossible to discuss how to improve your DNA without describing how to improve your diet. A key to this inner health is reducing inflammation. You can do this through cleanses on a short-term basis or you can start to maintain this type of diet day to day for long-term benefit. There are many great resources that you should check out, such as Dr. Alejandro Junger and Anthony William, who both speak about the benefits of a primarily plant-based diet in detail within their work. If you do want to continue to eat red meat in great amounts, I highly encourage you to read Shanahan's book, discussed above. She describes the four pillars of health and how to properly cook meat in detail. For the purpose of *Fertile*, I maintain focus on a primarily plant-based diet with healthy fats because it helps to reduce inflammation, enhances fertility, is non-harming and will raise your vibration.

---

21   (M.D. C. S., 2008)

A healthy digestion system creates a state of well-being, increased intuition and energy. Your gut works similarly to your brain helping your body to function. Ninety-five percent of the neurotransmitter serotonin is created in your gut, and a healthy system will help to protect you against suffering from depression. When our bodies become stressed, or we do not eat right, we will begin to show overt symptoms, such as irritable bowel syndrome, skin problems, weight gain, depression, headaches, fatigue or insomnia. You will not begin to know how bad you feel, until you know how good it can get. Eating the wrong foods on a long-term basis can cause chronic low-grade inflammation in your gut. In fact, you may be in a state of chronic inflammation and not even know it.

When your skin is inflamed, it becomes red and swollen, but when the immune system is mildly affected, you may not even notice it until it is too late[22]. Fatty or high carbohydrate foods promote inflammatory substances in the bloodstream, such as endotoxin, which leaks through the intestinal wall causing inflammation. This disturbs your health, specifically by affecting your blood sugar levels and your liver's insulin response. Junk foods, fast foods and sugary foods all have proven risks and there is a strong link between inflammation and chronic disease. This is worth paying attention to if you are going to bring life onto this planet.

Let me give you a few reasons that may motivate you to change your diet before you have a baby. Fetal Alcohol Syndrome was once thought of as unpreventable. It took doctors a long time to finally correlate the negative effects of drinking alcohol during pregnancy to malformations in the child. Cigarettes were once advertised as healthy and cool. Spinal cord and brain malformations were thought to be an accident until research found that folic acid (which had been depleted from the soil, thus affecting the nutrition in bread) could help to reduce the occurrence.

We were doing surgeries on infants without anesthesia up until recently. Our consciousness is not up to where it should be, nor is our scientific research. Many of the foods you are currently eating were not available for consumption even fifty years ago, and we really have no idea what they are doing to our systems.

---

22   (Tanzi, 2015)

I am going to postulate that many of the foods I discuss below will be deemed toxic during pregnancy in the future. You are just going to have to trust your gut that I am right on this, because I promise you that the companies that sponsor these items aren't going to research the side effects.

Sometimes it takes the government years to catch up to protecting society in the way it should. There are a lot of reasons why massive changes cannot be made because of the types of organizations that are actually in control of your mind and well-being. This is why change is very difficult in regard to gun control, cigarettes, tanning beds, or asbestos. Commercial interests often win over health and no one is going to put money towards studying the negative effects of foods that make large companies billions of dollars each year. The best thing for you to do is to remain informed and know how each item personally affects you. This can be done by eliminating them and feeling the difference it makes on your health, at least while you are pregnant. The good news about all of this is that genes are adaptable and we can heal. I am going to break down what you should and should not eat, especially during the delicate period of conception and pregnancy.

Vegetable Oil and Omega-Six Fatty Acids

Saturated fats and cholesterol are not problematic for the heart. The cause of health issues is due to processed fats, which are also known as Omega-6 fatty acids. These can be found in vegetable oils that are temperature sensitive and are extracted from corn, canola, soy, sunflower, safflower, grapeseed and rice bran. These products should not be heated, as the rise in temperature breaks up the fatty acids and creates a toxic effect on cells resulting in inflammation. The trend to fry fast food is relatively new and started around the 1950s. This change in diet has resulted in one of the leading causes of death and illness in Western countries.

Using vegetable oil on salads or for baking is also toxic. Even if you just consume a small of amount of trans fat, it can reproduce inside of you and form free radicals that damage and inflame your cells and arteries. Along with the oils listed above, Omega-6 fatty acids are also found in processed foods that use soy oil, appearing in grain-fed beef, meat of factory-raised animals such as chicken or pork, and non-free-range eggs[23].

Vegetable oil can affect and interfere with any cell in your body leading to all sorts of diseases. This is absolutely critical to understand when it comes to the development of the baby in the womb. Shanahan explained that studies have shown oxidative stress and disruption of hormonal responses to the fetus in women who consumed vegetable oil. It causes inflammation of the gut and negatively affects the immune system, causing nerve degenerating reactions. The more processed fats that women have in their diet the greater the likelihood of developing ovulatory infertility. These fats can interfere with ovulation, conception, and early embryonic development[24].

Do you have heartburn or digestive discomfort? This may be the cause and should be the first thing you eliminate. Vegetable oil is known to attack the brain and has been linked to autism and Alzheimer's. It can also impair brain development, altering DNA and genetic expression. Processed fats directly mutate DNA and make the genome more susceptible to environmental pollutants[25]. We have no idea the amount of damage it is truly doing to our bodies, because companies do not want to fund research that will show us.

Let me Break it Down for You

·   Good Fats: Olive oil, peanut oil, butter, macadamia nut oil, coconut oil, animal fats in normal proportions and flaxseed oil.

·   Bad Fats: Canola oil, soy oil, sunflower oil, cottonseed oil, grapeseed oil, safflower oil, non-butter spreads (margarine) and trans fat spreads.

·   Salad dressings: Loaded with both good and bad fats (read the labels).

·   Margarine: Interferes with normal bone growth.

---

23   (M.D. C. S., 2008)

24   (Chavarro, Willett, & Skerrett, 2008)

25   (M.D. C. S., 2008)

· Rice milk: Contains vegetable oil.

· Soy-based products: The processing of these packaged products damages the cell of the soy and has harmful effects on the body.

· Breakfast cereals: Most are coated with vegetable oil to maintain the shape — there is very little nutrition.

· French fries, cookies, and crackers: Full of vegetable oil and lack of nutrients.

· Granola, soft breads, buns, and muffins: Full of inflammatory trans fats.

Grains

Grains are toxic for most of us because we have not evolved to function on the grain-based diet of our present time. Albert Villoldo, author of *One Spirit Medicine*, explained that our ancestors ate a plant-based diet high in healthy fat. We lost the connection between Spirit and the natural world during the agricultural revolution, which was ten thousand years ago. Villoldo said, "During this time we switched from a fat-and-protein-rich Paleolithic hunter-gatherer diet … to a diet based on wheat, barley, rice, and maize — grains with a high glycemic index, or blood-glucose potential." When our ancestors began to live on this high glycemic diet of sugar, the centuries that followed were filled with war and conflict.

We are not presently eating the same wheat that people were given just seventy-five years ago. To eliminate famine, post-World War II, a dwarf wheat was introduced, creating twenty times more gluten in breads than older strains. Gluten is found in most grains including wheat, rye, and barley. The carbohydrates from grain break down into glucose. When we are fueled by a sugar-based diet, rather than a fat-based one, our moods and mental functioning are negatively affected.

There is currently a craze for eliminating gluten from your diet. From what I have seen, not everyone is affected in the same way from this product, and only a small percentage are truly allergic to gluten. It may cause some people to have stomach distention and gastrointestinal issues and others may not feel a thing. The only way for you to know the effect that gluten has on your system is to eliminate it for a minimum of two to three weeks and then consume it again to feel for reactions. I am not recommending that you stop eating grains entirely. The quality of the carbohydrates that you eat is what matters. Choose whole grain bread. Eat slow digesting carbohydrates such as brown rice, whole grained pasta, and dark bread.

Sugar

Villoldo explained that the typical American adult consumes one hundred and fifty pounds of added sugar yearly, including fake sugars and those in the forms of processed foods. Evolution didn't prepare our bodies for the heavy loads of these foreign foods. Imagine what we are teaching our children and how we are affecting their moods. Sugar is constantly being used as a reward for our youth and is also a form of emotional relief. It is one molecule off from heroin and stimulates the same receptors in the brain. Sugar is also one of the greatest addictions on the planet and it is the leading culprit of bad bacteria in the gut, and a sluggish brain.

The body knows sugar is a toxic substance: it jams hormonal signals, clogs up nutrient channels, and impairs mood and memory[26]. It also stiffens collagen in tendons, joints, and skin. This can cause arthritis and premature wrinkling. When it binds to hormone receptors and blocks them, it can make you insensitive to insulin, making you age and gain weight as you grow older. Do you suffer from headaches? It is not uncommon for people who have cluster headaches (often mistaken as migraines) to eat too much sugar.

The substance can damage brain cells and it is super addictive. Studies have shown that it surpasses the desire for cocaine with a high level of addiction matching that of the desire for heroin in many people. Sugar can increase the likelihood of diabetes, and if you have this disease during pregnancy, you are ten times more likely to develop a child with a major birth defect. Diabetes has a profound effect on prenatal growth. Even if you are borderline diabetic or insulin resistant you need to get this in order before conception.

---

26 (Villoldo, 2015)

The Truth About GMOs

GMOs are crops that compose more than seventy percent of the foods in American stores. The DNA of these crops has been altered to create new and stronger strands so that the products last longer and are resistant to pests in the field. Villoldo explained that ninety percent of the corn grown in the U.S. has been genetically modified by splicing in Bacillus thuringiensis (Bt) bacteria. The industry says that this does not pose a threat to us, yet studies have shown that Bt causes allergic reactions and intestinal damage to rats and farm workers who have been exposed to it.

Many supporters of GMOs have said that the crops would reduce the need for chemical fertilizers, increase yield, and be used to feed the world's hungry. So far this has not been the case, and many European countries have completely banned the products as they are yet to be proven safe. Independent scientists claim that they can cause food allergies, antibiotic resistance, immune suppression, and toxic reactions. The only way to know that you are not eating a GMO food is by buying foods that are "Certified organic by the USDA."

Roundup is another product to be aware of that is used on crops. It is a pesticide that is believed to alter the DNA of the friendly bacteria in your gut—even after you have stopped eating it. It is commonly found on soy and corn products around America. However, many organic farmers have reported that Roundup was found on their crops despite the fact that they did not spray. This is because Monsanto, the company that produces this pesticide, is not properly regulated in the U.S.—also the case of GMOs. It is important to encourage senators to mandate that independent scientific research studies be conducted on these issues in order not to remain victim of this type of massive food control.

Toxins and Heavy Metals

Anthony William, author of *Medical Medium*, was provided the gift to speak with Spirit in childhood and has since saved thousands of people's lives and improved their health through simple changes in their diet. William said, "If you're looking to point fingers about how things got so bad in the world, here's where to look: radiation, toxic heavy metals, the viral explosion and DDT." These invisible intruders have wreaked havoc on our health for decades or longer and are passed down through family lines. Even if you don't have overt symptoms of heavy metal exposure, you can easily pass these metals on to your children. I highly recommend that you do a heavy metal detox six months to one year before pregnancy.

It is important that men reduce their toxic heavy metal loads too, as mercury is one of the main causes of the drops in fertility in males. The specific protocol for doing this is in William's book, and it includes incorporating Hawaiian Spirulina, frozen wild blueberries, cilantro, garlic, and barley grass juice into the diet (William's explained in interviews that women can continue to eat these products to remove heavy metals while pregnant). Other supplements that are helpful to improve male fertility include ashwagandha, zinc (for healthy sperm), red clover blossoms, and vitamin B12. You can reference all of William's books for more information on improving your health.

Heavy metals are responsible for more ailments facing our bodies and our planet. Over a very short span of time, we have released thousands of synthesized molecules into our air including flame retardants, nonstick pans, plastic, and medicine in drugs. There is no data on the long-term effects of what these products can do to our health. Villoldo stated that there are eighty-two thousand chemicals approved in the U.S., and only a quarter of them have been tested. Most of these chemicals remain in the environment and affect our food. He said, "Because of the toxins in our brain and nervous system from pesticides and mercury, we can no longer readily experience unity with all creation. No matter how arduously we meditate …" The human brain is not designed to take on this type of toxic overload, and we need to be aware of what we eat, wear, and give to our children.

Dairy

Many conventional milk products such as cheese, yogurt, ice cream, and butter have been altered with a synthetic bovine growth hormone (rBGH). Some studies have linked rBGH to elevated risks of cancer. When cows are given this hormone, they have been known to suffer from shortened life spans, mastitis, increased birth defects, and high rates of diseases, infertility, and stress. Antibiotics fed to livestock can enter the human food chain, affecting the way hormones are metabolized in our bodies.

Dr. Christiane Northrup, author of *Women's Bodies, Women's Wisdom,* explained that women get relief from heavy menstrual bleeding and endometriosis when they stop consuming dairy foods. She saw in her personal practice a link to dairy and chronic vaginal discharge, acne, menstrual cramps, fibroids, and intestinal upset. She noted that the patients who changed to organic dairy products sometimes saw a decrease in these symptoms. Be willing to attempt to eliminate dairy from your own household for a couple of weeks to see the effect it has on your family. Milk is not the best source of calcium, and there are a lot of alternatives including increasing the amount of dark green leafy vegetables such as kale, collards, and broccoli. If you choose to eat dairy choose full fat organic options. Full fat products protect against ovulatory infertility and skim and low-fat milk products do the opposite.

Creating an Elimination Plan

If you desire to improve your health and upgrade your system before having a baby, you may want to eliminate some or all of these foods from your diet before conception. It takes about two to three weeks to fully eliminate a food. After this period, the best way to feel the effects is to bring one food back into your diet at a time. This way you can experience what each food does to your system individually, especially the effects on your stomach, skin and mood. If you can't handle a full elimination diet, try to take one of these foods out every week or two. Once you begin to see the health benefits of removing the inflammatory foods, you will likely want to continue making these changes.

It is especially powerful to detox and replenish the body in order to prepare for conception and keep your family healthy. This should go unsaid, but you must also eliminate alcohol and illegal drugs. You should not do a deep intentional detox within six weeks of getting pregnant. Never complete a heavy detox during pregnancy or while breastfeeding unless your doctor or practitioner says the supplements or foods you are eating are safe for your baby. Optimally create a detox plan and establish a healthy eating lifestyle six months to a year before conception. Make sure your eating plan meets all your nutrient requirements—especially proteins. When you are pregnant, please consult your doctor on how to maintain your clean lifestyle while still receiving the amount of nutrients needed to sustain your growing fetus.

If making these changes feels like too much, I encourage you to focus on just cutting out sugar and vegetable oils, especially while you are pregnant. The period is only nine months and it is totally worth it to protect your baby's health. If you cannot completely cut them out, at least reduce them. Absorb what you can about reducing the toxic overload in your body, but don't get too overwhelmed. Everything does not have to be given up at once. Small changes go a long way. Choose the alterations to your diet that work and go for it. Even buying organic or reading the labels and acting on the information can make vast improvements to your health. Reducing your toxic overload will help you to create a better brain and gut connection and ultimately more health and happiness.

What You Should Be Eating

Fat/Protein   Make sure to eat good fats: Omega-3-rich foods (such as wild caught salmon), avocados, nuts (no peanuts because of allergies), and coconut oil. Nuts and seeds are a good source of healthy fats and proteins. (Try soaking them for easier digestion.)

Fruit/Veggies   We co-evolved with plants, not with animals. Eat nutrient-dense, organic, and chemical-free fruits and vegetables. Include a lot of kale, collards, and mustard greens. It is ideal to have your diet be sixty to seventy percent fruits and vegetables. Villoldo explained, "A plant-based diet (nutrient-dense, calorie-poor) will switch on more than five hundred genes that create health and switch off more than two hundred genes that create cancers."

There is a high fear of fruit because people are afraid of sugar content and as a result they are ignoring the nutrient benefits. Anthony William predicted that in the coming years, scientists will create fertility drugs from fruit. He said, "Eat Fruit to Produce Fruit." This is very important. When you fill your body with high vibrational foods, the life-giving properties and energetics of the products become a part of you.

Adding plant protein instead of animal protein improves fertility. In fact, replacing twenty-five grams of animal protein with twenty-five grams of plant protein was related to a fifty percent lower risk of ovulatory infertility in one study[27]. Rather than eating a high-protein or a low-carb diet before pregnancy, focus on a natural glucose diet through organic fruit. Berries, especially wild blueberries, are excellent for balancing hormones. Other great fruits for fertility include oranges, bananas, avocados, grapes, melons, mangoes cucumbers, limes, and cherries.

Celery Juice   Celery is a powerful anti-inflammatory because it starves the bad bacteria in your gut. Disease comes from an acidic body, and green foods help to alkalize your system. Celery also helps to cleanse your body of toxic heavy metals. Drink eight to sixteen ounces or more of fresh juice on an empty stomach upon rising daily[28].

Fish   Eat small fatty fish, preferably wild caught fish, twice a week. Watch out for mercury toxicity. Small fish get mercury from eating algae and plankton. Bigger fish get it from eating smaller fish which causes a higher accumulation. Avoid eating fish such as bass, king mackerel, shark, swordfish and albacore tuna especially when you are pregnant because they are high in mercury, which can be toxic for the fetus.

---

27   (Chavarro, Willett, & Skerrett, 2008)

28   (William, 2016)

Eggs   Look for organic, free-range, pasture-raised eggs because they are higher in Omega-3 and vitamins A and E.

Breads   Make sure that you choose the whole-grain types.

Meat   Only free-range or grass-fed. If you choose to eat meat, you must know where it came from. Always trace your food back to its origin and understand the route of the source. Tracing the source of your food will allow you to better understand the types of nutrients you are eating and whether or not it is full of antibiotics or factory raised.

Supplements

The prenatal pill should be taken before you become pregnant, not just when you find out that you are having a baby. It benefits the first ten weeks of pregnancy and nutrients are needed for the baby's body to begin to be made. The prenatal pill is **NOT** enough to fulfill all the nutrients required to create a child and protect your own needs. Studies have shown that, despite taking a prenatal vitamin, women were still low in Vitamin D. Low Vitamin D levels in early life is linked to schizophrenia, diabetes and skeletal disease. Nor is choline typically added to prenatal vitamins, and deficiency of this nutrient is associated with lifelong learning deficits.

Vitamin A   Helps to regulate excessive estrogen levels.

Vitamin B12   Essential for liver detoxification and for protecting DNA. Most of us are B12 deficient. Be sure to take sublingual methylcobalamin, an enhanced form of B12 that dissolves quickly under the tongue.

Vitamin C   Essential for detoxification processes.

Vitamin D3   Can prevent or reduce depression, dementia, diabetes, and autoimmune disorders.

Folic Acid   Protects the baby's neural tube development. One study showed that women who got at least seven hundred micrograms a day of folic acid from their diet were forty to fifty percent less likely to have ovulatory infertility then women taking less than three hundred micrograms[29].

Iodine   A trace element that improves cognition, metabolism, protects the thyroid, and balances hormones. It is necessary for optimal health of the breasts, ovaries, and uterus.

DHA & EPA   Omega-3 fatty acids are important for brain health and preventing Alzheimer's. Take this in plant-based form.

Curcumin   The active ingredient in the spice turmeric activates the genes that turn on powerful antioxidants in the brain. It has mega anti-inflammatory effects.

Probiotics   Creates healthy flora in the gut and facilitates digestion. If you choose to eat dairy, eat whole-fat active yogurt which contains probiotics. An even better idea is eating probiotic foods, such as sauerkraut and pickles.

Iron   In one study, women who regularly took iron supplements were forty percent less likely to have trouble getting pregnant. The benefit came from these women taking forty to eighty milligrams of iron daily. The source of the iron mattered—women who got most of their iron from meat in the study were not protected against ovulatory infertility. Iron from fruits, vegetables, beans and supplements were beneficial to becoming pregnant[30].

---

29   (Chavarro, Willett, & Skerrett, 2008)

30   (Chavarro, Willett, & Skerrett, 2008)

A-Lipoic Acid Helps eliminate toxins and heavy metals in brain tissue.

Mg Citrate   Helps with your bowel movement and to eliminate waste; it is also a muscle relaxant.

Vitamin E   Helps to boost fertility and is a natural antioxidant. Take up to five to eight hundred IU for a few months before conception, as it helps the fertilized egg stay attached to the uterus.

Vitex (chasteberry) and ashwagandha are herbs and aptogens that can be used to boost fertility.

The combination of CoQ10, Vitamin D and DHEA is often prescribed for women with a low egg reserve (or a low AMH lab value) in fertility clinics.

Consult your doctor when taking any herbs, supplements, or vitamins during pregnancy.

Are you feeling overwhelmed or asking how it's possible to make these changes without going crazy? If you aren't ready for full throttle, my advice is to make one change every week or two and feel the difference that it makes. It's likely that if you drastically reduce everything at once you will feel overwhelmed and quit. Or cheat like I used to do. It took me a lot of time—in fact years—to really start to make huge improvements in my diet. I still have a treat here or there, but I am more cognizant of what I put into my body because I know the effects. When I am working with clients, I always tell them to make one change they can stick with, especially when it comes to doing something that they have never done before, such as eating clean.

Here are a few reminders of what you can do to improve the health of your gut:

+ Eat fiber, fruits, vegetables and whole grains

+ Avoid foods processed with chemicals

+ Ignore the middle aisles of the grocery store as much as possible

+ Take probiotics or eat foods like sauerkraut

+ Eat less sugar or share a dessert instead of eating the whole thing

✤   Avoid vegetable oil and refined carbohydrates

✤   Know the original source of your food—especially if you eat meat

✤   Always purchase grass-fed beef, or animal products without added hor-
     mones

✤   Eat organic as much as possible

✤   Avoid GMOs

CHAPTER 4

HEALING GENERATIONAL PATTERNS

Memories are Held Within the Physical Body

The experiences that you have in the womb and growing up create a platform for how you experience the world for the rest of your life. If any of these memories are negative or traumatic, and they are left unhealed, you could inadvertently pass this pain on to your children. Unhealed trauma can weigh you down for many lifetimes as they are passed from one generation to the next. This means that you could even be dealing with the trauma of your ancestors. Your past pain is important to understand and heal because it provides the best road map of what you truly came here to do. It shows you how to heal others that are in a similar situation or who have fought the same battles. Your trauma provides the path to your greatest acts of service on the planet. Follow your pain to find your greatest pleasure.

Children who experience abuse and neglect are more likely to suffer from mental health issues, such as anxiety and stress. This vastly affects their ability to move in the world and handle their careers, education, relationships or desires for illegal substances in a healthy way. As a result of the way that our subconscious programs itself, even benign events can register as trauma because of the power of perception. Under the same circumstances, another individual may flourish. This is likely a result of a combination of resilience, persistence, inner drive, connection to a higher source, destiny, karma, and their subconscious mind.

Whatever the form of trauma, it lives within the body and cells. When it is released, so is the memory. I remember working in labor and delivery one night and a woman in labor began to experience unprocessed traumatic memories of sexual abuse during the birth. She was so frightened that she was screaming, not necessarily from the pain of labor, but from her forgotten memories. This caused her to have a cesarean. The memories were buried within the energy of her second chakra and were retriggered through labor and the pressure of the baby on her cervix. Your memories are held within your organs and energetic centers. The way you were treated as a child will influence the way that you act and feel as you grow older. Your past events control your present and they physically weigh you down—until they are cleared.

I suffered trauma, but I was one of the resilient ones. I did not have the easiest childhood. Despite this, I persisted and moved forward with a strong internal drive and motivation. From what I have witnessed, through my own journey and through those of clients, trauma can either cause individuals to become slow, isolated and unable to make life decisions or push them to run through life with nonstop activity. The latter, my solution, occurs because individuals either consciously or unconsciously want to avoid their pain. The act of doing something outside of themselves doesn't allow them enough time to see that they are actually suffering inside. Both of these ways of being are a form of depression, and happiness is usually found somewhere in the middle.

Many of the women I have worked with, who suffered from a traumatic childhood, started to move through life faster than a freight train with the demeanor of a valedictorian. This changed when they faced challenges such as infertility or the after effects of becoming a mother. These events triggered a feeling of chaos and being out of control. The road to motherhood forced my clients to slow down and unwind in order to heal.

Most individuals are moving through the world while unconsciously suffering, not even aware of how unhappy they are. The unhappiness stems from past conditioning, attachments, projections, fear, and the tendency to self-sabotage. These patterns are really difficult to break because they live within the cells and create the energetic field. If you keep attracting the same experiences over and over, it is because you haven't changed your frequency - you have not yet healed the underlying belief system or pattern within you. Your mother and father have the same issues and as a result you created groups of friends, a career, a family, and a community all based on your past conditioning which was ultimately started in your mother's womb. This is why you don't know anything may be inherently unhealthy in your life, because your entire world mirrors your subconscious programming.

A somewhat painful event will likely have to occur in your life to deconstruct your conditioning so that alchemical spiritual transformation can take place within. Alchemy is a purification process that your soul goes through to mature and resemble its original nature. It is an esoteric experience that is unique to your personal path to awakening to a higher power. Spirit works directly with you via the elements to help you ascend and become whole when you are ready. This experience isn't necessarily pleasant, which is why many people avoid spirituality. The "pain" caused by this event is just your perception, but the discomfort is necessary in order for you to become aware that something needs to change. Until you fully awaken, you cannot see your life for what it is: a world where you are not in conscious control of your body, mind, or spirit.

If you were abused, neglected or felt unworthy as a child, you likely attracted a partner with the same tendency and you may be living your life replaying the same wounds. Beginning to see yourself - all of your flaws and all the ways you have not risen to your fullest potential—is the path of self-realization. Awakening is journey. It is a series of alchemical initiations. Consider the journey to pregnancy as an opportunity to rise to the occasion and change yourself for the sake of your entire genetic line. Your children will provide a mirror of your unhealed wounds if you do not, which is why I want you to clear them now.

The Research

There are many studies that demonstrate how negative experiences in childhood affect the demeanor and future of an individual. Growing up in extreme poverty early in life can cause a decline in physical and mental health later in life.[31] Emotional comfort is just as important as the safety felt through materi-al items or a stable home. A study showed that when monkeys were separated from their mothers and raised in cages, they developed severe detachment from their environment, hostility towards their own bodies and the inability to create attachments later in life. It makes me sad that we even have to test something like this. The consequences of a lack of loving relationships in childhood seem obvious to me.

Another study directly identified how maternal mothering can affect the epig-enome. After baby rats are born, it is normal for the mothers to lick and groom their pups. Not all mothers do this to the same extent though. One study showed that the rats who were birthed by mothers that spent less time licking and groom-ing their babies grew up to have higher levels of stress responses, a heightened response to stimuli, and were more fearful of their environment[32]. These rats were shown to have more methylation in a particular genome region of the DNA. They produced less of a protein that would have helped them respond to stress better.

Further studies showed that when rat babies were taken away from their un-maternal mothers and given to mother rats that were more likely to spend time grooming the pups after birth, they grew to be less fearful adults. Their experi-ence changed their demeanor. The studies showed that the rats who were cared for by the more attentive mothers were more nurturing themselves when they became a mother. A higher level of licking and grooming even influenced how the rats responded to cognitive tests for attention and spatial learning. The early environmental behaviors of the mother programmed not only the DNA, but the brain and intelligent responses of the animal[33].

Scientists have also shown that PTSD can be biologically passed down through generations. A study looked at eighty children with at least one parent who was a Holocaust survivor and compared each of them to fifteen individuals in a sim-

---

31   (Moore, 2015)

32   (Moore, 2015)

33   (Moore, 2015)

ilar demographic who did not have parents that experienced the Holocaust. The children who had parents who both suffered from PTSD after the Holocaust had higher levels of glucocorticoid receptor that helps to modulate stress response. Memories are often inherited and experiences that happened generations before can affect you later in life. Not only can your father's or grandmother's memory be passed on to you, but your personal memories can program your child in the womb. Your physical body is a hologram which stores all of this information. The denser the information, the denser the hologram.

Healing Through Alchemy

Unfortunately, it usually takes someone hitting rock bottom before they are ready to make changes in their life or clear limiting patterns, painful memories or self- sabotaging tendencies. For some, it is a lot easier to forge ahead and numb the pain on a Friday night with alcohol or drugs than actually deal with it. You don't know how bad it is, or how much better it can actually become, until you are forced to take a deep look in the mirror and make a change. You can continue to blame every relationship or person in your life for your issues, but it really has nothing to do with them. It is all you, love.

If you haven't had the chance to see how your past affects your present, this section should shine some light on this area for you. If you have tried to hide or ignore physical or sexual abuse, traumatic births, miscarriages or abortions (or anything that directly affects your body or body image), it is time to look at these wounds head-on. And even if none of this has happened to you, I know that you have a friend or a distant family member who has been affected. You have the power to heal this for all of these women and I will teach you how here. This work matters because until all of us are ready to rise up, there is still more work to do on Earth. My hope is that you can begin to see all your weaknesses and heal them for your children.

At some point in your life, you may feel the effects of alchemy, which is a force of transformation that happens in eight steps. When your life falls apart, or you feel some sort of a catalyst move through that forces change, you are likely in the first step of the alchemical process which is calcination. You may lose your partner, health, child, house, career or best friend. It feels like you are on fire and the entire world is falling apart. What is really going on is that you are physically changing to become more dynamic spiritually. Your ego is slowly being broken down as you continue to move through the alchemical process—or through the elemental forces of fire, water, air, earth, and ether, which purify you here on Earth. Alchemy is one of the fastest ways to God because it peels you open like an onion, exposing the parts of your life where you need to change. This process is your road to clearing generational history, trauma and heartbreak. It is the path to enlightenment and becoming a whole human being.

The alchemical process of transformation uproots everything you thought was safe and stable in your life. Almost everyone is continually experiencing alchemical changes, but not everyone is aware of this, nor is each person's level of transformation equal to another's. I am not going to go into the specific steps of alchemy in detail in this book because the breadth of the information is too substantial for the purpose of our work here. (It also needs to be personally experienced to fully comprehend the magnitude of the changes.) What I want you to understand is how the elements are an integral part of your awakening process. They can create balance or imbalance within your life and affect your fertility because they are connected to Mother Nature.

I am going to discuss each of the elements and their corresponding geometrical shape as they relate to certain physical issues that can be held within your body. If these issues are not healed, they will manifest and creep into every part of your life. They will also be passed on to your children, creating the belief systems and core components of their genome. The following information is based on the life work of my teacher, Celestine Star, my personal experiences and those of my clients. As you read about each of the elemental relationships, make a note in your journal of all the places where you recognize yourself or another person. Write it down, because I will teach you how to release it later.

The Effects of Unbalanced Elements in Your Body

I am going to use sexual abuse as a general example of how an event can create imbalance of the elements within. I chose sexual abuse because one in three women have suffered from this. You can replace much of the following information with whatever type of trauma or drama you have experienced, as it all affects the elemental and physical makeup of your life. Examples of events that physically affect you include sickness, pain, miscarriages, rape, surgeries, physical abuse or traumatic births. There are obviously many mental and emotional problems that are also held within the body, but here we will generally focus on the physical issues for the sake of simplicity. The effects of these events vary in intensity for each individual, but the physical density will always weigh you down. You will likely be able to see parts of yourself or another within all of these unbalanced elements discussed below.

If you have been sexually abused, there will always be mistrust of the perpetrator. Until you have healed, you will attract lower nature Beings and people into your life due to your feelings of being unworthy. If you were abused when you were very young, and never had a relationship before this encounter, you will always feel impure because of the loss of innocence at such a young age. You may continue to abuse yourself by sleeping with various men or being around men or people who hurt you.

You will inadvertently and continuously attract the people with the same vibration in order to relive the trauma in the hopes of healing it. This is something that you cannot stop unless you take time to recognize what happened to you. Unhealed trauma, or ancestral wounds, live within the subconscious and arise to be eliminated. Abuse can cause anger and may make you feel like you need to get back at the world, or at the perpetrator or the situation that caused you pain. It is critical for you to comprehend how pain experienced in the past can creep into the present moment.

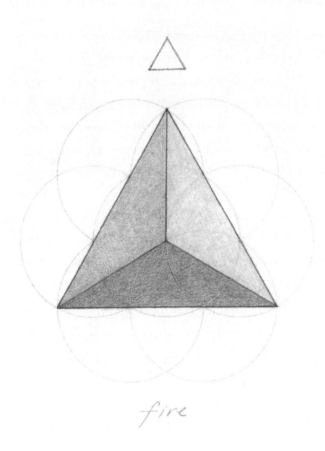

fire

Fire (Tetrahedron): This element represents the abuse or violence itself. It is a moment in time that burns the hole in your pocket which makes everything fall through. It is the opening of the legs or the taking from the womb. Fire is nature out of control. It is fierce pain that pierces your heart and soul or yoni. The flame burns continuously and anything that comes into your field will catch on fire too. You may attract very low or unconscious people so that you can burn them. This will help you to feel in control again or prove to yourself that you still have power. When this occurs, you know your fire is out of control. It is easier to see the weaknesses in others before we see it in ourselves: Do you have a friend that burns through partners or jobs? Do they partake in mischievous or self-sabotaging behaviors and not necessarily comprehend the damage that they have done to others or themselves?

An unbalanced fire element creates self-destructive and painful choices that hurt the individual and everyone around them. As you begin to purify, the salt of your tears will clear you and put the fire out. If you were sexually or physically abused, part of the healing is pushing off the perpetrator. You have to go back to the moment in real life and physically pretend that you are pushing someone away using, for example, a pillow. It is sometimes necessary to relive all the pain - physically feel and act it out—in order to burn it out of your system.

Going back in time and rescuing the inner child, who is still wounded, is a vital part of the healing process. You can actually locate your wounded child in your timeline and put her in a safe place surrounded by loving items and people. My inner child is living in Big Sur with a loving grandmother. She spends her days playing and gardening. Many people I know create a physical altar in their house for their inner child with toys and books. Taking the steps to heal your wounded child will help you to prosper in the present moment.

In order to heal, you can go through your memory bank and find all the painful events that are still hurting you. Take a sabotaging pattern, such as always being afraid that your partner is cheating and going to leave you, and find all the memories where you felt abandoned throughout your childhood. You can locate these memories within your chakras and organ systems by closing your eyes and scanning your body. These events may have a texture, color or shape. Energetically pull the memories out, relive these experiences in your mind's eye and, consciously using the element of fire, burn the whole story to ashes using your imagination.

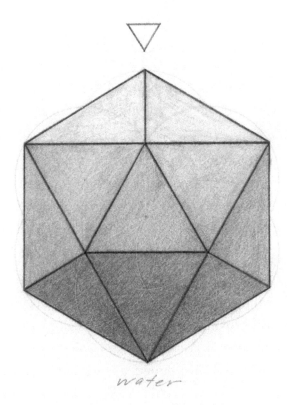

water

Water (Icosahedron): When the water element is unbalanced, it may feel like you are drowning in emotional grief. The emotions of suppression, depression and oppression are common. The element water is often pushed down because very few people want to talk or think about negative events from their past. The level at which this suppression takes place depends on their history and current environment. Water has the ability to hold the other four elements within it like a container. And if this container becomes unbalanced, aspects of all the elements may be released at once, causing havoc in a person's life if left unhealed.

If a person bottles up their emotions, they may become untrustworthy or delusional in their words or actions. They create internal and external illusions about the status of their life to themselves and other people to hide the pain.

This can come in many forms, such as acting like everything is alright when it is not in relationships, career or self-love. It could also come in the form of overbuying, overeating, overdrinking or oversleeping. These individuals are often embarrassed about who they really are and cannot face their faults, so they begin to tell lies that may be big or small.

I have a friend who was inappropriately touched as a child. Until she healed, she constantly felt all the unbalanced elements in her life, but the water element was particularly difficult for her. She drowned herself in alcohol in order to numb the pain and told lies to herself and other people to hide it. She overate and then submerged her head in a toilet to bring the food up. She created a front, or a barrage of stories, about how good she was doing externally, so that others could not actually see how bad she was feeling internally. Lies were so common that she got lost within them. As a result, she lived in the past or the future because she couldn't handle being in her present life circumstances.

If your water element is unbalanced, you may become a false storyteller. Truth will be difficult. Rampages of spending, drinking or drugs are not uncommon in order to hide or suppress the pain. If this hits home, until the tears flow and the truth is unleashed, you will be in a whirlwind of unresolved issues. You can alter the pattern of each element by mentally and spiritually using the element itself as the mode of healing. In order to heal the water element in yourself or another person, you can create an illusionary watery healing area, or even go to this place in real life. Water represents the subconscious and unconscious issues within you. At this water formation or lagoon, you can ask Spirit to purify you.

It is necessary to go through a purifying ceremony in complete sobriety and ask for all the unresolved issues to come up to be released. Within your home environment, it is also necessary to let go of any objects that are causing you pain. Put away the memorabilia of any family members or friends that you would no longer like to associate with, such as pictures or gifts. All of these physical items carry a vibration which affects you. This is the process of dissolution in alchemy, which is the letting go of outmoded belief systems or ways of living. As you heal, you must start on the path of total truthfulness. Be honest with yourself about what has happened and how you have hurt yourself and others by avoiding the pain. The ability to take responsibility for what happened in your past allows healing to rise to the surface from the depths of your soul. This is the beginning of spiritual maturity.

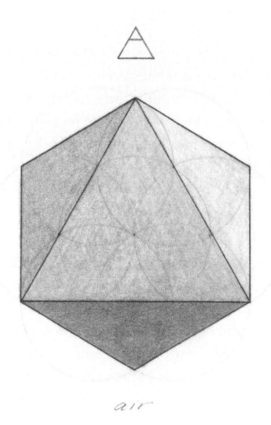

air

Air (Octahedron): An unbalanced air element creates a total whirlwind of a life. It makes an individual harsh and austere and can result in the loss of femininity. Have you ever seen someone who looks frail, tired, tight, or stripped of life force? Their air element is not in balance, which can make the heart shut down. The heart may feel like it is functioning energetically, but if your air element is out of balance, everything in your life will be done with practicality, total determination and a disconnection from yourself and others. You may feel a tremendous amount of vigor and the propensity to overachieve. This brings a lack of joy, natural flow and acceptance of what is. When you are always goal-oriented, it is hard to focus on the journey that gets you there.

Air can become hot and wound up, creating a vortex of energy that runs down the sacral chakra, or center of gravity and power. Women with unbalanced air may become activists because they want to fight. Wind is the element of anger and when it is not properly released, it creates inner turbulence and the need to be heard. Wind doesn't easily calm down and can be destructive to the environment around it. It causes individuals to feel constantly on edge and fearful about what will happen next. This creates a constant state of fight or flight, creating high cortisol levels in the body which decrease fertility. At its worst, unbalanced wind creates individuals who often have split personalities and a rollercoaster of emotions to counterbalance.

An unbalanced air element may create the constant need to control everything and everyone around you. This may show up in the neurotic tendency to clean, reorganize or constantly move around the house doing a lot, but not really getting much done at all. Control may come up in the areas of food, work, friendships, weight, money, sex, or love. In fact, control is one of the most common emotions that I work with within individuals who are trying to conceive. My clients who had controlling mothers or caretakers who controlled their childhoods often suffer from attempting to control every part of their process of becoming pregnant. The healing begins with the unwinding of both the tornado and the constant need to move forward with tremendous speed. The train must come to the station. You need to look at all the places you are wound up and tight, at everything you try to dominate, and all the ways that you can let go. Start with releasing the little things first. With this comes more spontaneity and joy.

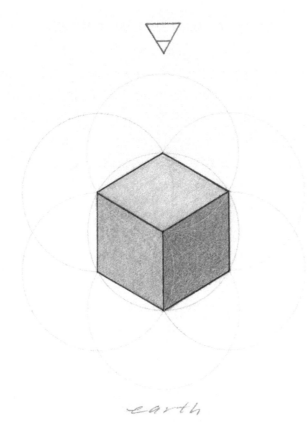

earth

Earth (Cube): This element can weigh you down when unbalanced. Reflect on what your life looks like—a good representation of this is your house. When you are spiritually developing, it is common to dream of houses in different forms, as these are representations of your physical and spiritual bodies changing. Is your current house dirty, cluttered, falling apart or in need of minor repairs? Do you move around a lot or miss your rent if you do not own your house? When your life begins to crumble, do you have the ability to build it back up just like you would a solid structure? If you have been abused, neglected or hurt, your earth element will not come together. You won't enjoy living in your own body and may dislike yourself. And your house won't be strong.

In order to heal, you have to look at all the ways that you need to rebuild your life. In *Mystical Motherhood*, I teach how to use Maslow's Hierarchy of Needs in order to become a fulfilled woman. This theory is applicable to healing the earth element. Start with ensuring that your needs of nutrition, sleep, sex, and shelter are met and then slowly move up the hierarchy into meeting the needs of safety, love, belonging and self-esteem.

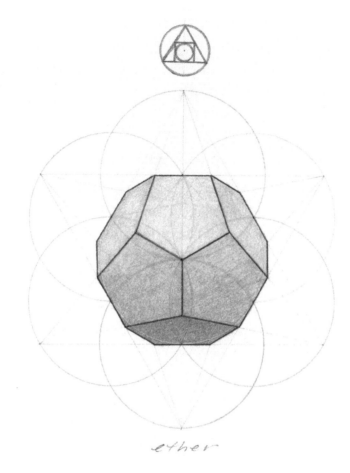

ether

Ether or Prana (Dodecahedron): When this element is in the destructive mode, it creates weakness and sickness. An example of this would be the cessation of your menstrual cycle. Ether works on your energy body and makes you feel powerless. Being exposed to pain or frequencies that are discordant on the inside will eventually weaken your immune system. If these painful experiences persist, they can break an individual down. When sickness and disease occur, it is a sign of the separation of the soul from the body or Spirit. You may not be able to make decisions because you feel disconnected. You may not even be able to dream because the etheric body has been torn.

If a traumatic event occurred and the person wasn't able to protect themselves, they may call on a protector. This can be detrimental, because the protector can be an outside source such as a negative spiritual energy. It is not uncommon for individuals who have suffered from physical, sexual, and mental abuse or alcoholism to have negative spirits attached to them. It is in moments of loss and desperation that a spirit will acknowledge a similar energy and attach. You can pinpoint when someone has a negative energetic spirit attached to them because they will suddenly change personalities. It is not uncommon for these individuals, who are otherwise caring people, to be cruel, mischievous or self-sabotaging for no reason, completely out of the blue.

They typically find a way to ruin something when it gets good, whether that is a job or a relationship. There will likely be issues of love and abandonment with all their relationships and a constant need to blame or project. Once love gets too close, they find a way to question it or push it away, which causes the other person confusion. These individuals will suck out your energy, just like a vampire, because it is necessary for that negative spirit to thrive. They basically turn their lives over to the spirit.

Trigger mechanisms are developed over time and the negative spirit becomes the individual's personal navigation system through life, constantly checking to see if their environment is safe. The person becomes incredibly sensitive to their environmental surroundings and may be extremely affected by sounds, smells or feelings. It is not uncommon for this individual to become isolated or hypervigilant of people and places. A lot of trust issues may arise because the person was so harmed by the original trauma.

If this feels familiar for yourself or another person, ask these questions: Do you sometimes not recognize yourself? Do you have moments of lost time? Do you have problems remembering what you said to another person even when they try to remind you? Do you often lose people or push them away? If any of these apply to you or someone close to you, there may be an energy attached that is breaking down the life force. Removing this type of energy cannot be done alone and requires help from an outside source. It is imperative to find out why the spirit attached in the first place and ask why they are still there. Oftentimes it is the individual who wants to keep the energy.

If you need help on your path to healing you can write in to: www.mysti-calmotherhood.com for further assistance. Either I will assist you or I will direct you to a person who is the right match for your healing process. Celestine Star is a powerful healer who can also assist you or a loved one through the process of alchemical transformation—her information is listed at the end of the book in the reference section. The exercises below are based on her work with clients.

Exercises:

Healing Your Inner Child: Learn to Mother Yourself

1. List all your traumas or dramas between the ages of zero and twelve (if your mother has told you stories about negative events that happened while you were in utero, list those too as they can be addressed in the same way).

2. Rescue your inner child and begin to mother her. This can be done at one age or multiple ages. You can find this child in any memories that still haunt you or in memories left unhealed.

3. Take some time to tell this child that you love her and she is not alone. Hold her and make sure she knows how cared for she is. You can even hold a pillow while doing this. Allow any tears to flow or screams to arise.

4. Go into the memory - the actual room of the trauma or drama—and pick up this child. Carry her out of the house or place her somewhere that feels safe and secure. Create a loving home for her and a place that you can return to in meditation. Make sure she has all the amenities to keep her happy.

5. Talk to the perpetrators or past caretakers - whoever it is that caused you pain. You must be the adult that shuts them down, because deep in the subconscious mind this is still happening to you in the present moment.

Whatever the subconscious mind needs to do in order to dissolve the issues, do it. Put these adults in parenting school, bring angels in to take care of them, take them to a healing place, put them in jail or take them to court. Do something in your mind's eye that releases the pain and creates justice.

6. By mothering yourself, you will become a better mother. If these wounds are left unhealed, they will creep back into your own experiences, triggering you while raising your children. The cycle stops with you.

Understanding Your Earthly Contracts: A Writing Exercise

1. Why did you choose this? Why did you choose the events in your life? Why did you choose your family? You shouldn't be shocked by these questions, as we are all the creators of our own realities for our greatest healing.

2. Close your eyes and go back to the time before you were born. Imagine yourself looking down from a higher dimension at your mother's womb. You knew what your life would be like as you looked at this family. You were attracted to your mother's frequency, but why? What would you learn through her? By choosing this family, you knew you would experience specific events that would physically affect your body, mind, and spirit in this lifetime—and you chose it. What have you learned since your choice, and what benefits have you gained from these lessons?

3. Ask yourself the following two questions about the people and the experiences that you have dealt with (you can do this with each significant experience individually):

4. *Was it a personal agreement?* This would mean that you have done this to others and need to have it done to yourself. Or you needed to experience this to heal it for yourself or for a generational line.

5. *Or was it a mission?* Meaning you chose your family or the experience so that you could understand the pain and help others. The mission is for everyone and for the ALL. You may go in and experience a rapist—the totality of the pain, the grief—so that you can be a healer and heal others. You need to feel the pain of humanity to be a true healer and be trusted

that you have the compassion and integrity to support others. You walk into the fire and then you come out as a diamond.

6. Once you know if it was a personal agreement or a mission, you can complete the following ceremony. Say these words out loud: "I hereby release my contracts and/or soul tribes (which is your family and friends) or attachments to these lessons." You can visualize the contracts between specific people and yourself burning up in a fire. You can also visualize cutting all the cords that may be attached between your bodies. After doing this, the dynamics of these relationships will change.

7. Acknowledge if your mother, father, sister or brother is your soul tribe — which is the group of souls that you may have spent many lifetimes with, learning lessons. When you are ready to move on to the next Higher Self, you need to let go of this tribe. When you let go, you will be ready to accept your divinity and be unified into the consciousness of all.

8. Create a symbol to anchor your new life. This is the first shape that comes to mind. Symbols are forms of energy and communication which allow Spirit to speak a vast amount of information quickly. Take some time to let it unfold around you.

9. Once you change these agreements, the world around you will change. Your world will rearrange itself to accommodate your new ideas about reality.

Doing this work is vital so that you can become an awakened mother. There is no need to pass these patterns on to your children. If you had a whirlwind of a childhood, would you want your children to experience any of this? I highly doubt it. As you do this work and release your past, make sure that all the healing is done from the level of your heart not just the head.

The Effects of Balanced Elements in Your Body

Fire: When the element of fire comes into balance, you will become a living expression of the God-force energy and an incredibly dynamic individual. The fire element has the power to harness the Kundalini life force. This brings a connected creativity and expression of divinity here on Earth through whatever medium you choose, including creating children. You will feel inspired, creative and motivated to complete what you came here to do. Your destiny becomes evident and easy to fulfill. You are no longer stuck in the mundane or repetitive.

A passion for life becomes evident and whether that is creating art, raising children or working, you will feel the drive, and what you contribute will feel worthwhile and valuable. Energy is abundant and focused. Charisma will help you to lead others because you are connected to your Higher Self and Spirit. When you get to this point, you have gone through the fires of transformation and you have watched many of your negative patterns and beliefs burn to ashes. A diamond has been created.

Water: When in balance, this element allows your emotional body to relax and expand. You will resemble a container—able to hold others with your open and expansive approach to life. By this point, you will know where you end and another person begins. Like the edge of a pool, boundaries become natural and they are there for your emotional safety. No one can take advantage of you now because you have released the contracts of obligation. This broadens your opportunities. Life becomes beautiful and it flows with ease. You are not afraid to show yourself or who you truly are inside. With increased emotional intelligence comes reliability. The more you trust yourself, the more others begin to trust you. As your mission on Earth begins to change, you begin to adjust to this with harmony.

Air: Rather than being an unpredictable tornado, the balanced wind element brings calmness and radiates assuredness. This is focused determination with power. You begin to see clearly all around you. Though pain is apparent everywhere, you now know how to focus on love. It is natural to surround yourself with individuals who are similar—in fact you couldn't have it any other way. Relationships have changed at this point and have more breadth and connection. Running away from your past and personal faults is no longer an option. You now stand tall and remain present with yourself, breathing in your body with fluidity. This calms your nervous system down, which lowers your anxiety and anger. There will be a truth in your words and a desire to lead and speak because others will listen. The balanced wind element brings strength, love, and an open heart to serve on Earth.

Earth: This element will keep your life and body grounded when it comes into balance. You will easily begin to build a solid house, career or family life. The earth element creates structure, which magnetizes opportunities to you. Whatever you choose to excel in becomes possible because your auric field is grounded into Mother Earth. You become a solid creator of your reality and easily attract the material or spiritual needs required for abundance. Your life will no longer be falling apart or crumbling in areas, because you have created a solid foundation within, which becomes apparent without. This is the element that allows you to ground Heaven on Earth.

Ether: This element, when balanced, allows you to work with the higher realms of reality with ease. You will become physically, emotionally, mentally, and spiritually attuned to consciousness and be cocreator of your reality in conjunction with God. The angelic realms, Ascended Masters and higher Beings all become accessible because you begin to match their frequency with your lighter energy and thoughts. Your auric field becomes strong because you have cleared it. You love yourself now. Others will reflect this love back. The dream world will be in alignment with your truth because you now understand the story of yourself.

When ether is in balance, you are connected to your Higher Self and begin ascending to the higher realms while still being a fully embodied human. When you begin to connect Heaven and Earth inside, or the lower and higher selves, everything becomes alive. Your entire reality becomes conscious; your senses are fully awakened. All known and unknown worlds around you expose themselves. Everything in your life becomes a form of communication like divine art. Anything is possible absolutely anything. And you have to trust yourself that it's all real. Once connected, you will begin to see that your inner world is directly connected to the outer world. All parts of the outer world then speak to your inner world. Our ancestors understood this. When you open up like an innocent child, you can return to wholeness. This is the path of the warrior, the truth seeker, and the lover. When your elements come into balance, you will attract a high vibrational child unlike any other.

EXERCISES

Build an Altar for Your Child

An altar is a sacred place you create within your home (I discuss this in depth towards the end of the book). You can build an altar that represents the kind of child you want to birth into this world. The altar should only contain items that have significance to you, and have been charged with purpose. It must also have a representation of the elements I described above. If you have suffered a miscarriage, a good idea would be creating a memory box, or altar, for the child. I often ask my clients to write letters to their lost children and keep them on the altar until they are ready to let them go.

Tap into Your Intuition

Throughout this book, I have asked you to tap into your intuition through feeling and visualization. If you feel lost and cannot figure out how do this, here is something you can do: Begin by sitting upright with your eyes closed. Imagine a beautiful place on Earth and begin to walk through this location in nature that you feel connected to. Feel the love for Mother Earth and all of nature. Then send this love through your spine down into the earth like a tree would plant its roots. Allow your energy to ground deep through each of the elements within the layers inside earth. Then think of the sky above and send your love from the top of your head into the sky. You can imagine a golden thread or rope rising out of your spine and connecting to the moon, stars or sun. Once you feel connected to Heaven and Earth, tap into your heart and womb center by taking a few very deep breaths and visualizing the organs.

Creating a Family Tree

This meditation may take you days to weeks to complete. It is a process that can be continually worked through as you finish the book.

Imagine a cube. Visualize all the corners and lines of this three-dimensional square. This cube is clear and as you look into it, you see that it is split into three cross sections. There are two solid breaks in between the top and the bottom. These three sections represent your past, present, and future. As you look at your past, which covers the bottom of the cube, it is likely to be dense and darker in color. The middle may be lighter, representing the present, and the future is clear. Now imagine yourself holding this cube in your palm and then set it in front of you on a desk or table.

Bring out your journal and begin to write about all the issues from your past that create the density in your cube, any issues in your present that need to be resolved, and discuss in detail how you would like your future to look. This can be done in bullet points under past, present and future sections. Try to get as much done as you can in each sitting. Symbols, such as the cube, carry a lot of information and are a way that the Universe can speak to you. As you are writing, make sure to continue to go back to your cube in your mind's eye and ask your body to connect with each area of the cube fully. Ask for all memories, patterns, dysfunctional relationships, pain, and negativity to come up, in order to be released for the highest good.

Once you have this all written out, you will want to take this information and create a family tree to see if you can trace the core problems back to the generations that came before you. Take a concept or painful experience that you wrote down and have been holding in your body. Trace it back in time. Begin by writing down anything from anxiety to miscarriage to start. Ask your Higher Self to tell you if anyone else in your genetic history has experienced this. There will likely be an immediate knowing.

Create lines out to the people in your family that had the same problem occur to them. You may hear "Grandma" or "three generations back." Whatever you feel, hear or see around each of the issues—write this information down and learn to trust yourself. Ask for a higher source to come in to keep you open to receiving. You can do this for all the information you discover about yourself in this book down to the tiniest details, such as: weight gain, bulimia, reactive behavior, anger, depression, sadness or compulsive reactions. You may need a large piece of paper or a lot of space! That is totally normal, we all have a lot of history to let go of.

Know that by doing this, you are likely the first person in your family to even acknowledge the pain of the past and heal it into the future. When you do this work, you become the record holder and the healer for the whole family. It will all end with you, because of your dedication to create a better world. There is tremendous power in forging ahead into a whole new future for your blood line.

After you have written down any information that has arisen intuitively about issues from your past as they relate to yourself and other family members, you may want to reach out to family members to verify what you have found. Let me provide an example for you. I was working with a client that continually miscarried, and I intuitively knew that she had a family line of women who had the same problem which could be easily linked to her grandmother on her mother's side. She felt that this was correct too, and asked her mother about it—sure enough it was. Knowing this, she began to understand that she was repeating a pattern that went back in time through her family. She committed to healing herself from the inside out and the miscarriages stopped. Families hold secrets: admitting negative traits is a sign of failure. You will be surprised by what you find hidden within your genetic line.

A Meditation for Alchemical Transformation

Now that you have a larger picture of your own issues, and an intuitive sense of how these issues run back through your DNA and past generations, we are going to work on healing them at a spiritual level using alchemy. The elemental process of alchemy will transform and alter your life. You will need to be alone in a room for a period of time for this next part of the process.

Create an altar with the five elements in front of you: a candle that is lit to represent fire, a glass of water, a representation of air such as a feather, a piece of nature that represents earth and something representing the higher realms for ether. This outer ceremony will help you transmute on the inner realms. Before you begin the following visualization, you may need to connect to Heaven and Earth first as described earlier under *Tap into Your Intuition.* You will also want to ask your Higher Self that all records from your past be opened in order to be healed for all past generations. You are asking to help transmute your genetic line and release that which no longer needs to be passed down—for the benefit of all and the children that will be birthed through your womb.

Close your eyes and see the Family Tree you created above drawn on a piece of paper in your mind's eye. Under it is a golden bowl, representing your womb. Imagine that the ink with which each of the issues has been written is dripping like water—dripping into the golden bowl. Each problem is being released.

As each issue drips like tears falling, allow memories to arise. Screaming and shouting are welcome. There may also be flashes of insight from your family history. Don't be surprised if you feel hot, cold, sad or angry. Allow it all.

Ask your body to begin to pull out all of these memories from your cells and imagine these memories are going into the bowl too. It may make it easier if you say this command out loud: "I am clearing (insert memory) from my cells and DNA."

Once this history has been wiped clean, and you have felt the emotional, physical, and spiritual aspects of all of these memories, all your genetic information will be held in the element of water within the bowl.

In your mind's eye, hold this bowl high with both of your hands and ask a higher force, such as Mother Mary or the Holy Spirit, to help you transmute it into gold. Ask that the energetic contents be released. To help you do this, visualize a flame that is blue at the bottom and red at the tips burning the bottom of the bowl, heating up the water.

As the flame burns, it removes the blood line and memories. Visualize DNA being cut and put back together into its most crystalline form. This clear and crystal DNA will run throughout your body soon. Let this flame burn as long as needed to fully remove all the pain from your physical body.

Just as Jesus turned water into wine, watch as the water in your golden bowl turns red representing your DNA in its purest form. As the contents continue to heat up you will begin to see evaporation rise representing the transformational power of the air element.

When the element of air has cleared the contents of the bowl, you are left with the pure salt of your tears in the shape of the cube—your soul's essence. Visualize the cube you began this meditation with, now completely clear. Pick it up and see it as a three-dimensional representation of your cleared genetic and generational history. This cube represents the earth element in its most refined state and at its highest frequency.

Place this cube into your uterus or womb, asking your body to keep this sacred shape safe until you conceive your child. If you are already pregnant, ask that the current child be cleared. This cube will help to anchor this higher vibration into your body. Allow this clear cube to become the frequency of a magnet attracting a powerful soul or keeping your current child safe.

MIND — THE TRIANGLE

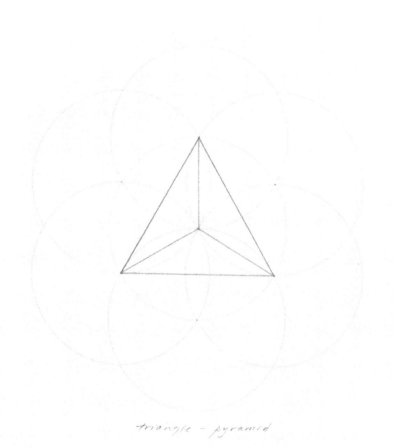

triangle — pyramid

CHAPTER 5

MASTERING YOUR MIND

The human mind is a very powerful tool. Your thoughts can be your worst enemy or best ally. While you are reading and interpreting the world during pregnancy, you are simultaneously programming your baby. Each of your thoughts creates a hormonal cascade and emotional waterfall that affect your growing child. It is possible to create an experience of love and harmony within your womb even if your life is not going smoothly. The perception of your environment and how you react to it is what matters. You can consciously design what type of child you are creating during this sacred period of growth by choosing better thoughts and mental projections.

Your mind writes the screenplay creating the drama of the movie that is your life. Your thoughts create the framework for the characters, circumstances, and choices that star in this modern-day drama. Until you choose to change the underlying story line of your screenplay you will be playing the same movie on repeat your whole life. (The film *Groundhog Day* is a good example of this.) When you are pregnant you can imagine that the womb is one large cineplex movie theatre. Whatever movie you are playing in your mind during pregnancy will program the consciousness of your child. All of the details of the screenplay that your child watches matter and your level of consciousness is the child's only reference point. Each character, scene, and line of the movie are creating the fetus's view of the kind of world he or she must be prepared to live in.

If a horror film plays a couple of times during pregnancy, your child has the resilience to handle this. If this film is on repeat, the tragic outcome is a child who is prepared to survive in whatever type of movie he or she experienced while living in the womb. My goal is to teach you how to play mental movies based on love, belonging, and harmony so that we can create higher vibrational humans. It is time to clear your generational programming, to take back your power, and get in control of the way you perceive your world in order to create a child that can change this planet. Whatever you broadcast to your baby creates the chemistry of their blood. You are the genetic engineer for your child. What type of individual do you want to birth?

The Subconscious Mind

There are many facets to our minds, but the two divisions I will discuss here are the conscious and subconscious levels. The conscious mind is controlled by Spirit; it is our true identity and is full of expansion, connection, and creativity. The subconscious is more like a garbage dump made up of memories from our childhood. Bruce Lipton referred to the subconscious as video tapes of our life that we recorded up until the age of seven, whether they were good or bad events[34]. The subconscious is our reactive mind that moves from instinct. When it starts getting full, it will unload into the unconscious. This then enters the conscious mind which is your waking world.

When this happens, you suffer nightmares daily. The subconscious mind holds all your memories, events, patterns, and beliefs that you may not even know exist. When these are not released, they will overflow to other parts of our lives, creating neurosis, obsessions, depression, or negativity. When you are so full and heavy, you can't help but repeat the same mistakes, thought patterns, or language throughout your life. This is why releasing negative thoughts, generational patterns, and belief systems is so important. It is also the reason you should start a meditation practice. If you don't know where to start, there are many Kundalini Meditations as taught by Yogi Bhajan, specific to pregnancy and motherhood, which you can find in *Mystical Motherhood*. These meditations will help you clear

---

34   (Lipton PhD, 2015)

programming from your childhood so that you don't pass it on to your children. I will teach you more about this later in the chapter.

Ninety-five percent of the time, you are being controlled by the subconscious programming you received from your parents or caretakers[35]. The largest portion of this programming was done in utero. As a woman, you can clear hundreds, and even thousands, of years of history by approaching motherhood with a higher level of consciousness. Until you realize that you are repeating the same patterns passed down from one generation to the next, you will be living like a zombie, or a character in a movie, playing a predetermined role. It is time to wake up. When we fail at something, such as giving up sugar or losing weight, we tend to blame some outside source for our own self-destruction. As a society, we are completely unaware that our subconscious is running our lives and that the majority of these programs are disempowering, self-sabotaging, reactive, and negative.

Humans can choose to react or not to outside stimuli. We also have the power to change old programmed responses at any time we desire, once we begin to deal with the subconscious mind (which can be done via meditation, healing modalities, self-reflection or Hermetic schools). Let me give you an everyday example of this. My grandmother is terrified of cats. Probably at some point in her life, she experienced something negative around these animals, yet she cannot remember when or why. As far as she knows, she has never been physically hurt by the animal and there is no logical reason for this fear. It is just her belief about cats that make them scary. This same example goes for snakes or spiders or anything else in your life that triggers you (such as family or friends). If you are uncomfortable around these creatures (or people), you could make the conscious decision to change and just accept them as they are. It is only your belief that they are frightening which makes them so.

As the screenwriter for an epic drama called "creating life," choosing to include positive thoughts and uplifting emotion in your script means you affect the DNA of your baby in the womb. Even if you are in negative or stressful circumstances during pregnancy you can choose to react to your environment differently. I will

---

35   (Lipton, 2018)

teach some ways to do this towards the end of this chapter. By sending thoughts, messages, and mental projections based on love, rather than fear, you can create a higher caliber child. If you want to create a family that is different, and a child that is genetically original, you need to begin to think and perceive the world in a new way.

Behavioral Epigenetics and Blood Chemistry

Remember that a gene is just a blueprint that makes a protein. These proteins give us our physical assembly. Genes have no individual level of intelligence and your genetic history does not control your life. As the contractor and manager of your genetic profile, and that of your incoming child, imagine you are in a room full of blueprints. You can pull these pieces of paper out of storage at any time for modification in order to create a new readout or better design. There are many ways to alter your original blueprints; these include healing modalities, healthy food, peaceful emotions, mindfulness, immunity through increased health, decreasing stress, and being in relationships that bring harmony and peaceful environments. All of these experiences stem from a mind that can skillfully manage negative and positive input and project a life of happiness and abundance.

Let's go back to Bruce Lipton's research in the petri dishes mentioned towards the beginning of this book. He took genetically identical cells and put them into three different petri dishes containing a culture medium, which is a laboratory version of blood. When he changed the chemistry or composition of the culture medium (the blood), the cells changed. The chemistry of your blood controls the fate of your cells. The chemistry of your blood is created by the chemistry in the brain. All of the cells in your body are controlled by your thoughts. The pictures in your mind create complementary blood chemistry in your body through hormones or chemical messengers. If you are creating positive and harmonic pictures, you release positive chemistry. If you have fearful or negative thoughts, you create negative chemistry[36].

---

36   (Lipton, 2018)

The blood that feeds the placenta is not only bringing in nutrition—it is also delivering all the information of how the mother is experiencing the world around her. If the mother is living in a peaceful environment, she will support positive growth. If she is living in a world full of fear or stress, her blood chemistry will naturally complement that experience. In the womb, the baby is being pre-programmed by the mother's viewpoint of the world. Her attitude will prepare the fetus to survive in the environment that it is going to be born into.

If you feel loved and supported during pregnancy, your body produces the hormones dopamine and oxytocin. These create internal harmony, health, and vitality which help to enhance the intelligence of the child by routing blood to the forebrain of the fetus. A peaceful world will help to produce a forebrain that is highly conscious. If you interpret your world as supportive, a loving child will be born through the creation of a resistance-free environment.

If you are stressed, your chemistry releases adrenaline, norepinephrine and cortisol, which create a state of danger or threat. Stress activates the HPA system, also known as the fight or flight system. When this occurs, blood is routed to the child's arms, legs and hindbrain, ultimately creating a fighter or a warrior capable of reacting quickly in an environment based on survival[37]. Avoid emphasizing protection and fear during pregnancy, because these emotions create the fight or flight response and a negatively heightened gestational experience.

A few stressful events during pregnancy are not going to harm your baby. The goal is to not repeat the negative events, thoughts or emotions. Repetition is what creates learning patterns. If you are consistently projecting negative thoughts, riding an emotional rollercoaster, suffering from addictive behaviors or actively putting yourself in negative situations during your pregnancy, you are training your child to perceive the world in this manner. If you can devote at least one year of your life (the time before conception and during pregnancy) to mastering your thoughts, you will change your genetic history and every generation that comes after you. Remember, all major patterns and characteristics are established in utero. Your ancestors, and all the angels and saints, will be cheering

---

37 (Lipton, 2018)

you on as you endeavor to do something completely unique on the planet, which is breaking up the matrix.

Most of our world is in survival mode, living on the vibration of stress and producing a blood chemistry that negatively affects the immune system, thus creating disease. The sickness in our world is personally experienced by billions and manifested on a global scale through crime, wars, and destruction. You clearly know what you are up against, but you also understand that you are one of the people who volunteered to do it differently—otherwise you would not be reading this. Our personal consciousness is connected to the collective consciousness. It is necessary to dedicate time to your personal healing in order to clear yourself. If you begin this journey before conception, you will be in the window of fertilization that will powerfully and positively affect the egg.

Genomic Imprinting Before Conception

Ancient cultures, such as that of the Aborigines, had a pre-pregnancy cleansing period to get the mothers' consciousness to a level to accommodate their babies'. They honored their future children by purposely creating a higher level of consciousness and improving their minds and spirits before conception[38]. Modern scientists call this period of time *genomic imprinting*. It occurs when the activity of specific groups of genes are adjusted that will have an influence on the child to be born. The egg is susceptible to imprinting two to three months before fertilization. If you want to prepare your mind, body, and spirit for conception, this is the minimum amount of time that you would ideally plan for. You can do this for each child and even if you are already pregnant, it is never too late to start.

Epigenetic imprinting modifies the readout of genes within individuals. Nature doesn't determine the character of a baby until just before conception. Even though all of your eggs were produced years ago, what really matters is your level of consciousness at fertilization and during pregnancy. Our goal is to remove any negative imprinting from your egg, and this can be done by increasing consciousness through elevated environments, thoughts, emotions and even food. The way

---

38   Lipton, 2018)

you experience life in the period before fertilization will affect certain genes. This is also true for your partner. As a couple, if you create a calm and stable environment before conception, you will positively affect the genes of your offspring. If you continue to do this while the child is in the womb, you can help the child create a positive personality, balanced emotional temperament, and higher thought patterns.

The child you create will complement the environment it was created in. Environments have a dynamic effect on genes, even before conception. What you perceive, whether inside or outside, is who you are. You can structure your DNA by balancing yourself internally and externally. Everything has an energetic vibration, and if we want to raise ours, as humans and as planet, we must pay attention to everything in our environment on all levels. This entire book (and *Mystical Motherhood*) is dedicated to helping you elevate your consciousness, modify your genome and bring calmness into your life for motherhood. This is all in dedication to the sacred soul you are bringing in.

Eliminating Negative Beliefs During Pregnancy

When you begin to recognize that your thoughts and belief systems control your waking world, you can become the commander of a new reality. Now that you are aware of your subconscious programming, you have the opportunity to stop the generational patterns and not pass on outdated beliefs to your children. Your negative belief systems, which are both personal to you and similar to the collective, take up most of your waking hours and waste your energy.

Some common thoughts in women include I am ugly, all men avoid emotions, my mother is mean, everyone abandons me, I am unworthy, I am fat, everyone else has it better, you have to dress sexy to attract men and women are competition. When you think these thoughts during pregnancy, you are programming your child in the womb with the same defeating patterns. Can you imagine telling your baby that he or she is fat or useless? I hope not, because those are not nice things to say to anyone. It is vital that you become aware of just how vicious you can be with yourself, so that you are not in turn critical towards your child. We don't need to pass any of these negative beliefs on in the womb. These random thoughts keep you running in circles, while manifesting the same types of people and places around you.

Think of beliefs as folders on a desktop held within your consciousness. For each belief system, you can open a folder and find pages of memories that prove it is true, even when it is currently false. When something negative occurs, or you feel bad about yourself, you may recall that it happened in 1992, 1994, 2006 and 2013. Knowing this, you will then project that it will happen again now or in the future—probably again around 2033? This creates a negative loop and self-sabotaging patterns. You are constantly perpetuating cycles of repetition in your life because few of your thoughts or experiences are unique.

Let's break down the belief "I am unworthy" to find out how it is held in place within your subconscious mind. When you are not hired or do not become pregnant as expected, your consciousness will go straight to that I Am Not Worthy folder, pull out material and say, "See? Look at this! I have proof of what a loser I am. Look at all these other times I failed. I have never been worthy before, why would I be deserving now?" You then design your current reality to match this belief system and the cycle repeats itself.

If you are feeling bad about your body, your subconscious will pull out matching files to maintain your thought patterns. Your mind will create a stream of memories of all the other times you didn't feel good about yourself (... like that time in grade school when your mom told you to slow down on all the food you were eating or that other time when your college boyfriend looked at you funny when you took off your clothes ...). The mind likes to prove its points to itself in order to maintain control. Your subconscious constantly works behind the scenes as a twenty-four-hour detective and lawyer who defends the ego.

This is all really disturbing, because none of these stories are true. You may think they are because you are constantly recreating them in the present moment, but I promise you the opposite can always be proven. Think of the world as one large holographic computer. Other people are mirrors of your personal insecurities, fears, and negative thoughts. Your original holographic nature matches that of Spirit or God. When you are full of subconscious junk, and undirected thought patterns, you will create human drama. It is all a play and you write the storyline. Recognize that your mind is the main hard drive that can override the matrix and all your personal negativity. This is your power.

As a mother, you could potentially pass these negative patterns on to your baby, but with conscious intention you have the capability to transcend your thoughts. When the neutrality and awareness of your mind increases, the polarity on the planet will not affect you. Recognizing the positive and negative of each situation is a critical skill to have because these concepts help you to form neutrality, or a mind stream connected to God. When you are connected to this higher consciousness during pregnancy, you are programming your child with divinity, rather than your personal human story. Meditation and focused intention will help to get you there. Through a dedicated practice, you can choose to step out of your personal drama and alter your child's destiny.

Recognize Your Life Themes and Mental Intrigues

Start to make a list of everything that you have a tendency towards repeating in your life that is negative. This may include issues around your self-esteem, anger, depression, addictions or relationships. As you become more aware, you will likely see similar themes. Your mind is a recorder. When a habit enters the recorder, it will begin to automatically play itself back through your behaviors, feelings, and thoughts. Be honest with yourself and recognize that a lot of these issues bring you down and take away precious energy.

When your mind is not neutral and clear, you suffer from brain fogginess, self-defeating patterns and what Yogi Bhajan, the Master of Kundalini Yoga and Meditation, calls mental intrigues. These intrigues create every kind of thought—positive, negative, mixed, contrasted, reactive, and projective[39]. None of these are accurate because they are not from Source, Spirit or God. While you are riding a roller coaster—going up, down and all around— you are also most likely creating unnecessary guilt and feelings of being limited and inferior. Your mind is vast. When thoughts are intently focused upon, feelings arise. These thoughts and

---

39   (Bhajan, 1998)

feelings then build upon each other creating imagination and fantasy. The situation becomes intensified and the mental intrigues create unhappiness.

Without a clear relationship with your mind, your ego will begin to take over. The ego loves to create complications in your life and when it becomes afraid, it starts to exert power over situations and people. Individuals use emotional responses to control others when their ego feels threatened. This is a vicious cycle that can be subdued through an active awareness of your thoughts and themes in your life and integrating meditation into your day. Here are some ways to become aware of your mental intrigues or life themes, which are repeating events.

✤ Identify your mental intrigues: The first signal that demonstrates that you may be caught up in a mental intrigue is when you feel that you cannot handle a situation. Your body may be in one place, but your mind is in another. When your mind begins to go very positive or negative and you become obsessed with something, this is when you need to start to pay attention.

✤ Locate your themes: Life themes come in all forms and are backed up by your thoughts. You may tend to have the same fight with different people, leave jobs, eat too much, always run away from problems or relationships, repeat the same negative words, or consistently pick the wrong friends. Once you locate your themes, choose to become actively aware of them. Say to yourself, "OK, this seems to be a theme and it doesn't make me feel good. I am going to start to pay attention to where else this pattern exists." At this point you should be really excited. You discovered it!

✤ Notice your emotions: Each theme or mental intrigue in your life is connected to an emotional response and there is always an emotional reaction behind the pattern that will set you off. If you ever have trouble locating your life themes or mental intrigues, pay more attention to your emotions. You can follow each emotion back to the thought. This is when it gets good because you can then choose a better one.

✤ Become neutral: Begin to watch your life themes and mental intrigues. This is a huge step. Knowing that they exist and becoming a neutral observer of your negative habits is essential to the steps necessary to change them.

✤ Then ask yourself: How can I start to change this negative theme? You can begin to neutralize each theme second by second by sitting with it. Breathing deep into the moment and recognizing that the same pattern is repeating itself. A simple example would be criticizing your partner by picking out all the things they do wrong rather than what they do right. When this habit starts to arise again, notice it. Instead of speaking negatively in the moment, sit with it and take seven to ten breaths. See if you care anymore.

✤ Acknowledge your past: You may want to locate all the places in your life where this pattern has come up before. Themes extend back to your childhood and create looping thought patterns. Maybe your mother criticized you and possibly that is why you tend to be critical towards yourself and others. Do not go into victim mode when you start to look at your themes. You do not want to open up Pandora's box and create a story that may start looping towards your mother. Just softly acknowledge that this has happened before and now you know why it may be happening now. Be gentle with yourself. No shame or blame.

✤ Train your mind: Your goal is to create a relationship with your mind. When you start to go down the rabbit hole of mental and emotional despair, talk to your mind. Tell it that you are the Source of God. You must actively engage your mind to create a relationship to it. It takes time and motivation to excel.

✤ Become aware of yourself: You need to start a meditation practice. Meditation is not an option anymore—it is essential. There is too much pressure in this world, and a state of neutrality amid the chaos is vital. It will help you to continue to find your patterns. You are your own worst nightmare. The only way to control your subconscious thoughts, which control your daily life, is to make meditation a part of your routine.

Meditation is Your Saving Grace

Just like you take a shower and brush your teeth to clean your body, your mind also needs cleaning. When you do not meditate, the power of your subconscious and thoughts will entrance you. Getting caught in this downward spiral makes individuals feel small. As a result, they attempt to expand themselves through outside sources. Anything that pushes individuals up and out of problems, such as drugs or alcohol, is only going to cause more issues.

Analysis or psychotherapy is helpful to reveal issues, but it is not a long-term solution. A lot of our issues are buried deep in our subconscious and we don't even know that they exist. Many women who were sexually abused can't even remember what happened until they go through therapy. Analysis should be used to understand your history and identify your problems, but if you continually go back, you will likely create more of them. Your mind will mentally loop your past problems into current relationships because you will be constantly talking about them. Your words and thoughts create your reality. Be careful what you say.

Kundalini Yoga and Meditation, as taught by Yogi Bhajan, is the fastest growing yoga on the planet and also the fastest way to increase awareness. It cuts to the chase by diving directly into your subconscious programming and removing it. This ancient Indian yogic system is a science and technology that balances the pineal gland, glandular system and hormones so that you can choose higher frequency thought patterns. The meditations are generally active with movement and mantra or sound currents, which makes them fun.

Meditation creates a habit so that you are able to sit with your mind in order to review it and direct it. By choosing better thoughts you will create higher caliber experiences. As I mentioned previously, I dedicated my first book, *Mystical Motherhood*, to teaching this ancient science along with a step-wise approach to improving your family throughout motherhood. The *Mystical Motherhood* website contains free meditations to download and information to read with step-by-step instructions on the history of this yogic lineage, how to start a practice, and specific meditations to use throughout your journey. If this specific kind of meditation practice does not feel right, I encourage you to research other forms of mindfulness, healing techniques or yogic practices.

How to Rise Up and Create Boundaries

When making life changes for personal well-being, resistance may arise at any time. I know that most of our histories make it hard to overcome our patterns and neurotic tendencies. I also know that there are legitimate painful and stressful experiences that can arise at any moment such as a death, divorce, job loss or family dynamics. Life isn't always a breeze and our minds can easily get carried away with how difficult things are. One of my teachers taught me the following Yogi Bhajan quote, "Let the whole world fall, but not *insert your name here*." Now, say this out loud three times.

This is the type of assertive energy you have to maintain when you are protecting yourself and your baby from outside programming. Mama Bear knows best. You must trust yourself and know what types of people, places, noises or activities will trigger you. Avoiding external stress whenever possible will help you to create internal mental peace. If you want to keep your mind neutral, it may be necessary to skip certain experiences that tend to upset you while you are trying to conceive or are pregnant. During this sacred period of time, your peace and harmony should be an absolute priority.

Sometimes you may need to make boundaries in relationships that are hurtful to you, cut back your career stress if you can afford it, or choose to go to a meditation class instead of a loud restaurant. Every experience that you have will directly correlate to the level of consciousness you are programming your eggs or baby with. In order to keep your frequency high, it is necessary to pick higher vibrational people, places, and activities. This may require cutting out poor life choices or negativity for a period of time. Choosing to consciously spend your energy focused only on elevating yourself could change your entire pregnancy.

I work with many women who have issues with fertility. We address healing their problems around control, family trauma, and specifically their mother wound. In order to be in control, they have to let go of it. Control appears in various forms: a packed schedule with too much time dedicated to family and friends, issues around food, addictions, traveling and work. When there is not a balance between doing and being, your body and mind will build up tension. Conception, pregnancy, birth, and motherhood are enhanced through relaxation.

I worked with a woman named Jessica: she realized just how rigid she had become in her thinking and life. This stemmed from the need to demonstrate perfection to her parents with the best grades, dating the captain of the baseball team and a perfect body. This rigidity created an eating disorder and the inability to let go of toxic relationships and negative work situations. When she began working on herself, she distanced herself from her mother in order to reflect on the relationship, and not get triggered. Creating this space for healing vastly improved her current relationship with her parents and the boundaries she needed to make with them before starting her own family. At work, she learned to say no to staff who were not the right match to work with. She made boundaries with friends who were no longer making her feel happy, and she looked deep into her issues around food and perfection.

Jessica had to let go of everything in order to gain everything. She learned to trust and let Spirit guide her. She had been taking the prescription drug Clomid to increase her fertility for six months, and her doctors recommended in vitro fertilization. The treatments made her feel crazy and gain weight. Her mind was out of control with thoughts of depression and worthlessness. I recommended that she get off all of her medications and allow her mind, body, and spirit to heal. I told her to give it three months and she would be pregnant.

Despite having irregular and lengthy menstrual cycles, while what I said was against all medical advice, she listened. Intuitively she knew that she couldn't enter pregnancy in such a chaotic mental state. We used the *Mystical Motherhood* protocol and dove more deeply into all of the issues discussed above. Jessica maintained an active Kundalini practice using specific meditations aimed at increasing her fertility. Three months to the day she was pregnant. Jessica healed and has delivered her first child. She gained a clearer mind and a highly conscious approach to motherhood and life in general.

Though many of my private clients have become pregnant naturally as a result of this work, I also practice Western medicine as a Nurse Practitioner at a busy urban fertility center. I know that many women require medical help with conception. I understand the stress that these women face and I hope that this book can relieve some of those feelings. *Fertile* is not necessarily a guidebook to help you become pregnant naturally. The intention of this book is to help you become a better mother. No matter how you become pregnant I want to relieve your stress so that you have a better pregnancy.

In fact, I believe in creating harmony within so much that I recommend the following: if you have been having trouble conceiving and feel completely crazy as a result of the pressure the experience creates, seek medical help at a fertility center. If you are under the age of thirty-five and have been trying to become pregnant for a year or you are over the age of thirty-five and have been trying for six months, you should seek help. When you do, try your very best not make yourself feel bad about it. There is a lot of shame around infertility in our society that I hope to decrease here. If you require procedures such as in vitro fertilization or intrauterine insemination to become pregnant that is alright. Make boundaries for yourself on how much stress you can take during this process and learn to accept help. Spend your time working on your mental, emotional, and physical well-being instead, so that you can enter pregnancy in a state of love.

What I am teaching here is interdimensional midwifery. You are the gatekeeper between worlds and it is an honor to hold your hand through this process. You have a powerful role on this planet and can make magic happen. Jessica's story isn't going to be everyone's, but I can promise you that if you do the work you will become a better human who will create profound human beings. If you have had babies before and didn't know anything about the material in this book, don't worry! Neither did I and my babies are "usually" angels. Do not feel any guilt for what you did not know in your previous pregnancies. You know better now, and can utilize this knowledge to help yourself and all your friends. No matter how long it takes you to become pregnant, or whatever stage of motherhood you are in, the work you do to internally balance yourself is going to pay off.

The Pictures in Your Mind Program Your Child

Slipping away from the stress or drama may not be an option for you, or anyone. I want to offer you some coping mechanisms to handle these life adversities through the power of your mind. If you remember anything from this book, this is it: *when you are pregnant, it is your perception of your environment and how you react to it that matters, not what is actually going on around you.* I have presented this before, and it bears repeating. Your mental projections and level of consciousness are what will be broadcast to your child. Even if you are in the midst of family chaos, you can actively choose to maintain images and feelings of love and harmony for your baby. The ultimate goal is to broadcast higher thoughts in order to maintain a peaceful vibration.

Every individual has a different reaction to stress. Some people can handle a storm and walk through tornadoes without getting lost in mental intrigues or emotions. Other people must monitor their surroundings and maintain simplicity in their life in order to keep it together. If you are in situations that you just can't get out of, I want to give you some skills to handle your thoughts. My background was difficult and I have had tragedies throughout my life that have brought me spiraling down. I know it requires resilience to make it through difficult experiences. Motivation to grow and neutrality also help. The key to handling stressful events is to ask yourself the following questions:

- *Am I accurately seeing the other person's perspective? Do I understand how the other party may be viewing this situation and how they are affected?*

  - Knowing the answers to these questions will give you a wider perception of the event and a sense of neutrality.

- *Is this experience as bad as my mind is making it out to be, or am I getting myself caught up in a negative loop?*

  - If you can find something that you appreciate about the situation, you will begin to change your thinking and gain your power back. Appreciation holds a very high vibration.

♣ *Do I have enough energy to get myself out of this?*

· Negativity thrives on repetition and it takes energy to get from the negative mind stream to a positive one. You can gain this energy through meditation, mantras or exercise.

♣ *How often am I repeating this story out loud to others in order to find justification that I am right?*

· We all want to have a bigger experience of what we are feeling inside, whether it is good or bad. We often repeat our dramas out loud to different people for justification or solace. This in turn perpetuates the mental projections.

♣ *Am I able to see the opportunities for growth this life situation may be offering me?*

· For every negative experience, there is an equally positive viewpoint. What if you chose to focus on what this situation is offering you instead of remaining the victim? Taking a different point of view could change your mind.

♣ *Is this thought form worth my time and energy? Is this something that I would want my baby programmed with?*

· This second question is probably the most important one. If you can't stop the negativity for yourself, at least try to do it for your child.

When I was interviewing Bruce Lipton to complete this section of the book, I asked him how women could potentially program their babies and just how powerful the images in our minds are. He gave me an explanation around food as an example. He said that it is not necessarily the food that we eat that matters. It is our thoughts around the nutrition in the food, and our overall outlook on health, that will create an impact on our bodies and level of consciousness.

Obviously, we should eat clean and healthy ingredients whenever possible to counteract negativity, but it is the images in our mind regarding our health that affect our nutritional input. Lipton said when you have a picture in your mind of what you are creating, your digestive tract will remove specific nutrients from your food to manifest that image for you. This is how powerful you are. If you are mentally creating the image of health, your consciousness will do everything in its power to assist you to maintain it.

Belief systems are powerful and create your life circumstances. There are some groups of people that drink poison and do not die because they hold the belief system that they cannot get injured. Other individuals believe they can live off air and sunlight and they do. The placebo effect is an excellent example of the power of our minds. Sugar pills have demonstrated time and again that they are just as powerful at healing as medications, because it is an individual's belief system about the pill which creates the healing.

During the period of conception and pregnancy, you must cultivate a mental picture of health and well-being. Higher frequency thoughts and feelings are based on love, harmony, acceptance, appreciation, trust, beauty, truth, peace, and reverence for God. If you aren't feeling well, or your emotions are negative, check what is on repeat in your mind. Do whatever is necessary to reverse these mental patterns using any of the tools mentioned in this chapter. Your reactions and your perception of what is happening around you are both a reflection of your current level of consciousness and your determination to choose a different thought. As the genetic engineer, artist, and screenwriter for your child, I encourage you to create a masterpiece.

CHAPTER 6

CREATING THE HOLY TRINITY

The triangle represents the diamond facets of the mind, but it also creates the Holy Trinity. For the purposes of *Fertile*, the Trinity is the relationship you have with your partner and the divine energy that the two of you create together. It is the representation of the holy mother, holy father and divine child, which is an aspect of the Holy Spirit. If you remain in balance and in synergy with your partner, the combination of your frequencies will create an enhanced unified energetic field. This third field is a subtle and palpable energy of love that can be directly transmitted to the creation of a child. Though there are many types of unions on this Earth, here I will focus on that of a man and a woman and their ability to consciously conceive in a heightened sexual union and healthy relationship.

A couple who creates a direct connection to Source through a partnership that is based on love, harmony, trust, and conscious communication will live within an enhanced energetic environment that will ultimately attract a high-caliber soul. This type of partnership has the potential for improving your cells and DNA because it brings great joy. I believe that as infertility rates rise in the future, the couples that are in balanced union will have fewer issues becoming pregnant. A cosmic sexual, mental, and emotional connection between a man and a woman may eventually be a necessary component for conception through intercourse. Internal balance, and the lack of physical and energetic density, ultimately creates a fertile atmosphere. When an environment of heightened love and support continues throughout pregnancy, couples will program their children with these same dynamic traits.

When an individual is in union within themselves, their masculine and feminine qualities are in harmony. They are whole within and do not enter a partnership with the hopes that the other will complete them or meet their personal needs. Individuals attract partners with similar energetic signatures or lessons to work out together. Relationships create a mirror that reflect where you need to grow. Essentially, within a divine union, the personal mirrors have been cleaned so that each feels union with God through the reflection of the other's eyes.

Components for the process of creating a holy child are the relationship you have with your partner, the type of energy the two of you create together, and your ability to connect into higher dimensions to create light—especially while making love for the purpose of conception. Men and women who have done their personal work, who are in touch with their higher selves and are connected to Source, create a new frequency together. Their connection is both seen and unseen. A dance of the soul where two become one. The two complement each other and aim to expand upon strengths rather than focus on each other's weaknesses for continuous growth. A divine couple has a specific energetic frequency, balanced elements, and complementary sacred geometry within their fields.

At conception and throughout pregnancy, the cells of your baby form sacred geometrical figures within your womb for the purpose of creation. I believe sacred geometry is the ancient secret to creating a holy child and that you can enhance the geometry of your child through your journey to higher consciousness. I am teaching you various ways to improve your body, mind, and spirit so that your cells and DNA will be amplified and the geometry of your child in the womb will be energetically cleared.

In order for you to understand just how important geometry is to conscious conception, I will take you on a journey back into the ancient times of the Goddess Isis. By becoming acquainted with her, you will meet the original genetic engineer of the planet and understand her part in the story of creation. I will also discuss how this Goddess and her sacred partner Osiris, along with many other divine couple archetypes, set templates for the ultimate sacred union on the planet. The interweaving of these subjects will eventually lead you to an understanding not only of how to create a deep love and connection with your partner, but also of critical issues to work through, with the goal of conceiving a child consciously.

(A note to the reader: In this chapter, I discuss conscious conception between a man and a woman. The information is still valuable no matter what your sexual preference is.

If you end up conceiving your child via intrauterine insemination or in vitro fertilization, this chapter will still be beneficial in helping you to maintain a loving and intimate partnership & to create a happy family.)

Sacred Geometry and Your Auric Field

The architecture of your energetic field or aura is created out of sacred geometrical patterns. The best reference I have for this is the famous drawing of Leonardo da Vinci's The Vitruvian Man. Leonardo's drawing of a man in perfect proportions demonstrates universal and cosmic design. The variations of sacred geometry within the human auric field correspond to the individual's level of consciousness and vice versa.

When your frequency is high, and your elements are balanced, you will create a geometrical field that is connected to Source or God. Just as you are not a victim of your genes and can improve your well-being and destiny on Earth, you also have the capability of altering the original geometrical design that was given to you by your mother at birth to create an advanced auric field which holds many gifts. And, as an engineer of your own child, you can also improve the sacred geometrical design of your baby during conception and gestation.

The Goddess Isis and Ancient Geometry of the Womb

Sacred geometry is a critical component to creating a holy child, as it is the basis of the Universe and our holographic nature. Everything in this world can be linked back to geometry. I previously discussed the development of sacred geometry in the womb upon conception and into pregnancy. Your DNA is made of sacred geometrical figures, and specific shapes are closely linked to creating a high-caliber soul (some even compare these advanced geometrical shapes to the creation of the Christ Child). *Fertile* is divided into the three sections of the square, triangle, and circle because these are the primary shapes that make up the most complicated universal structures.

When I was asked to write *Fertile* during a highly charged spiritual experience, I was given these three shapes in my mind's eye as guiding posts as to where to start. I did not know that these shapes would eventually reveal the role that sacred geometry and mathematics play in the creation of a child and the enhancement of DNA. Since my experience, these symbols have unfolded into a wealth of knowledge to help you learn how to enhance your consciousness with the purpose of becoming the conscious genetic engineer of your child, just as the high priestesses were in ancient times. When the square, triangle, and circle are energetically cleared, the DNA is enhanced along with the overall level of the consciousness of the human. I will discuss this in more detail as we move through this chapter. First, I want to give you some historical perspective of sacred geometry and how it relates to conscious conception.

When I began to write this book, a year and a half after receiving the three shapes, I took a journey through France where Mary Magdalene spent time after Jesus was crucified. Many people have an inaccurate interpretation of Mary Magdalene and do not know her as an ancient Egyptian Priestess, wife of Jesus and incarnation of the Goddess Isis that she was. I did not realize it at the time, but while in France, I was traveling over one of the largest temples created in the world covering over forty square miles of land. This temple layout, which was mapped via satellite technology, creates a sacred geometrical design representing the womb via mountain ridges, stones and churches. Over the centuries, this was both constructed and protected by the Knights Templar and Cathars. Both groups vowed to protect the Holy Grail and the secret that all religious organizations have tried to keep a secret: that the feminine was once worshipped as the creator of our world.

David Wood spent his life researching the sacred geometrical shapes that were left within the land of France and described his work in detail in the book *Genesis: The First Book of Revelations*. I highly recommend that you find this book if you are interested in further understanding the Divine Feminine, the Holy Grail and the origins of our species. Wood devoted his life to exploring how the mathematical layout of the structural sites on the land in France was linked to the creation of the human race as we know it. What he uncovered is far beyond the breadth of this book, but I want to summarize a few vital points.

According to Wood, after the floods of Atlantis (which covered most of the Earth and eliminated most of the population) the Goddess Isis was a savior of humanity. She, along with her counterparts Osiris, Set, Horus, and Nephthys, helped to regenerate the population of Earth and left evidence of how they did this on the land in France. This land is geographically in close proximity to where Atlantis sank into the ocean. You don't have to embrace the story of Atlantis to understand the purpose of why I have included Wood's interpretation of our history. The land carries the three geometrical shapes critical to creating the sacred child. Within this temple complex is a large rectangle which holds the other shapes—a five-pointed star (pentagram) and a six-pointed star (the Star of David or Mer Ka Ba), which are both made up of triangles. These shapes are held within circles. These figures have specific mathematical equations, which create the basic geometry found in the womb.

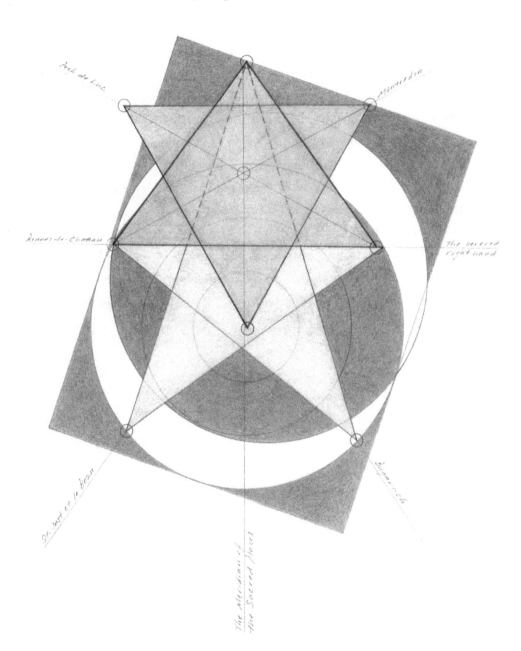

Mathematics: A Template for the Holy Child

The secret to this geometrical design on the land in France was repeating numbers and mathematics. Wood explained that when Isis created the species, she made man with the body of a beast and the mind of God. This was shown through the repetition of the number of the beast—666—which was depicted through the pentagram star embedded in the temple complex. The numbers 666 are representative of the fallen nature of man or individuals who are separated from their Source. Those who carry solely a 666 frequency may live their life without Spirit or God. The representation of our connection to God is the Star of David or Mer Ka Ba found on the land. This geometry includes fifth dimensional geometrical figures and symbols that have been used throughout history in reference to higher levels of consciousness.

pentagram

The Goddess created a beast with a mind that has the ability to function as God or the Universe, without the instruction or timeline to learn how to properly use it. She constructed humans who did not know how to effectively grow into the high level of awareness. To this day, we are still at this same evolutionary level on Earth. As we can see clearly from the state of our planet, this has led to great destruction of Mother Earth and has lowered the level of consciousness on the planet.

There was something hidden within Wood's book—a secret to creation that the Goddess left for us to uncover. This is the number 888 (the number 8, and variations of it, are connected to Isis). I believe that 888 is represented by the geometry of the eight-pointed star or the Star of Isis. Note that the number of the physical world is six and the number of the spiritual world is eight. The Star of Isis represents the symbol of the Rose and you will soon read how important the Rose line of women on Earth is to creating the enlightened child. You can use the eight-pointed star (Star of Isis or the Rose) as your energetic symbols in your journey to increasing your fertility.

Interestingly, when comparing this shape to the original geometry found on the land in France, the primary image is the pentagram with a secondary image of an eight-pointed star. When the star of the beast (666) is rotated (imagine turning it to create one more triangle), it creates the Star of Isis (888). You have the power to raise your vibration in order to transmute the pentagram into the Star of Isis or Rose within yourself, for yourself, and for the purpose of creating an enlightened child. The geometry is interchangeable. You can energetically rotate the pentagram in your womb. If there were a Star of Isis (rather than a pentagram) and a Star of David geometrically created in your womb during gestation, you would essentially be producing an entirely different type of human—one connected directly to Source. The eight-pointed star is a part of the sacred geometrical configuration that can be created within the child's blueprint when you complete the inner work of preparing your body, mind, and spirit for conception. By energetically clearing yourself, you will enhance your DNA and the sacred geometry of your offspring, creating an entirely new mathematical configuration within your child.

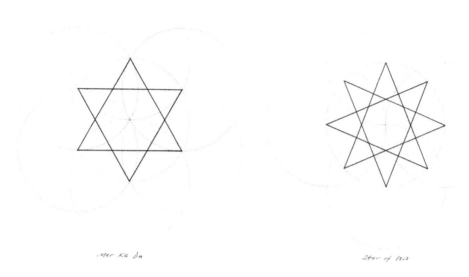

Mer Ka Ba   Star of Isis

The numbers 888 represent Jesus, the spiritual son (or sun) of God. Pythagoras' theory demonstrated this through a formula which connected the spelling of letters to numerical values. Those who hold the frequency, or geometry, of an 888 will have the mind of Christ. They have the ability to tap into the mind of God. These individuals live their lives much differently and carry a specific harmonic frequency that can touch into higher realms of consciousness and light itself.

The son of Isis, the God Horus, also held the archetype of the solar child who had gifts of utilizing the science and "harmonics of light." Pay attention to the words "son" and "sun." Ascended Masters, such as Buddha and Jesus, were "enlightened," which means they "move into the light" and carry the light of God within. They become one with the light of God. Later in the chapter I will go into greater detail of how to create this energy of light during sexual intercourse with your partner and how it has been done throughout history within sacred marriages. When a man and woman come together in balance, shining their own internal light, they will be able to touch into higher vibrational fields while here on Earth and make miracles happen.

A note to the reader: You don't have to believe that the Goddess Isis was the original genetic engineer of humanity if this challenges you. Consider the concept as another story of creation. Rather than using the word God as creator, this version uses the word Goddess. These words are actually interchangeable anyway. The main takeaway is that there is a blueprint held within your womb at conception and during pregnancy. The basic structure of your baby is the sacred geometrical DNA template that can create an enlightened child or not. It is important to mention the Goddess Isis, along with many other divine feminine figures in our history, because they also left us with a template of how to interact with the masculine in synergy and love. The love between a man and a woman helps to create the Holy Trinity or divine child. The Goddess Isis is also the representation of the line of women who hold the secrets of the Holy Grail.

The Order of the Rose and Magdalene Line of Women

The rose is the symbol of the line of women who represent the Holy Grail on Earth. It includes many divine feminine archetypes including Goddess Isis, Mother Mary, and Mary Magdalene. Though these women walked the Earth as mortals, they were also divinely in tune. They were all trained in ancient Egyptian sacred practices and knew the secrets to conceiving and birthing holy children. They, along with their sacred partners, left a template for us on how to do this. These priestesses delivered a code for fertility that we are unravelling here.

The Order of the Rose, a very ancient and secret order, is still present on this planet. This rose energy is asleep within the DNA of many women and is waiting to be reawakened in harmony with the rise of the divine feminine on Earth. This line of energy runs through women in the physical form and is also symbolically represented by the serpent (Kundalini energy) and Grail or Holy Cup. Women of this order will self-identify within their lifetime. They will know at a soul level that they are a part of this holy lineage because of their strong ability to navigate the inner planes of existence and higher spiritual essences on Earth. If you have an association with the Magdalene Order, you may be one of these women and it is not an accident that you are reading this book.

Members of the Order of the Rose have the inherent ability to awaken those they come into contact with just by their presence. These women also have the internal knowing of how to bring enlightened children to the planet because of their ancient Egyptian training from past lifetimes. There was also training for divine birth that was practiced in the temples of ancient Greece that some women may be attuned to. Their genetic inheritance, as we saw earlier, will naturally create the sacred geometry of the eight-pointed star (representing the Rose) combined with the Star of David or Mer Ka Ba (the six-pointed star) in the womb.

In order for this to happen, the women will go through a massive awakening process within their lifetime to fully identify with their divinity and raise their vibration to this level. These initiations are not for the faint of heart, and to call them "challenging" would not give them the respect they deserve. They are both an internal and external energetic experience created by the divine. For these select women there is no other option. They chose within this lifetime to undergo a spiritual death and resurrection in order to remember who they are.

If you feel drawn to ignite this genetic inheritance within yourself, you may consider traveling to sacred regions around the world that carry the frequency for your remembrance. France is located on the Rose Ley Line. This is an energetic Earth line representing the Goddess which starts at Rosslyn Chapel in Scotland, extends to Glastonbury in England, runs through Mary Magdalene's land in France and continues through the Pyramids of Giza in Egypt. If you are interested in reclaiming your divine feminine, and picking up lost pieces you left for yourself, I highly recommend that you visit these potent and activating sites. I was naturally drawn to visit these areas before I understood any of this, and the lands ignited the memories required for me to write this book for you.

Mathematics, Geometry, Music, and Harmony with Your Partner

The entire Universe is based upon mathematical patterns. Everything can be expressed through numbers that correspond to vibrations. Names, geometry, birthdates, and even your destiny can be linked back to numbers. These values are a critical component to creating sacred geometry. Linking these two systems—numbers and vibrations—becomes both a form of divination and magic

as mysteries unfold. Metatron's Cube unites the numbers six and eight because it
has six sides and eight corners. As you may remember, from the beginning of the
book, Metatron's Cube holds all of the platonic solids within, which make up the
sacred geometry of you and your baby.

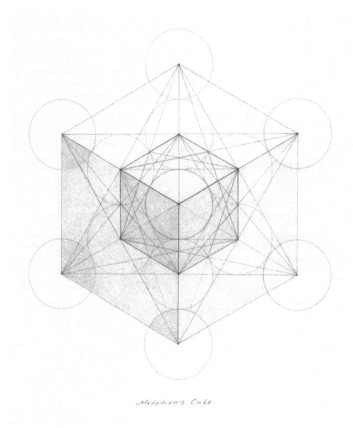

Metatron's Cube

As mentioned earlier, the platonic solids also have elemental attributes to them
(see the next figure). Not surprisingly, aspects of the platonic solids and elements
are also linked to the male, female and child. The tetrahedron (fire) and hexahedron (earth) represent the male aspect (left column of the figure). The dodecahedron (ether or prana) and icosahedron (water) represent the female aspect (right
column of the figure). The sphere (or void) and the octahedron (air) represent
the child (middle column). Microscopically, the dodecahedron and icosahedron

create the blueprint of life or DNA. These six shapes and six elements create a trinity of polarity.[40] Each of these are critical components of consciousness.

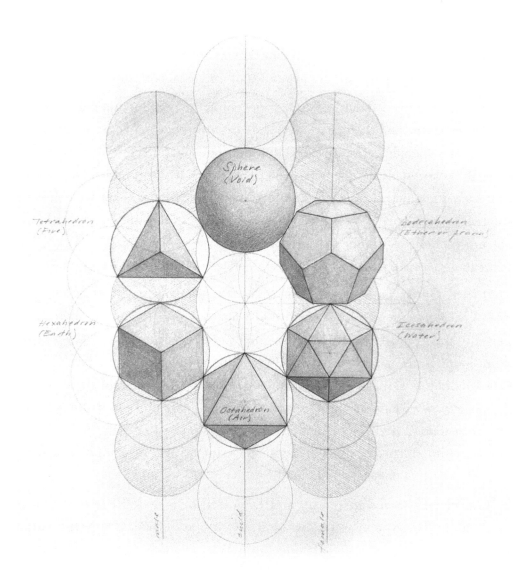

When these parts of yourself are balanced, you will naturally create the Holy Trinity within: a divine connection of the female, male, and spiritual aspects of

40 (Melchizedek, 1998)

God. This is connected to the number eight as a symbol of infinity. The human body is a hologram and contains the platonic solids within its field. You are a microcosmic representation of the cosmos. If you are holding a higher consciousness, not only will your elements be in balance within your field—in a natural dance of alchemical union—but your masculine and feminine qualities will also come into alignment. When this happens, you are whole, matching that of your Source, and echoing the sweet harmonics of universal consciousness.

Pythagoras unveiled many secrets concerning the relationship between music, sacred geometry, and the genetic code. He discovered that geometry and mathematics carry specific harmonies. The numbers 666 and 888 contain musical tones. Over the years, many people have used his research to continuously demonstrate that sacred geometry, especially the platonic solids, carries a harmony linked to the twelve-note scale. When specific points of the triangle are connected to create an icosahedron, which consists of twenty triangles, a natural three-chord note is created. Geometry carries a sound and since you embody it, you do too.

DNA is sacred geometry, so because of this we can assume that it sings. By now, I hope you clearly understand that your thoughts, emotions, environment, and diet affect your DNA. You can essentially create a unique sound or harmonic vibration in your cells and genome by making simple lifestyle changes. That is how multidimensional you are. Balancing your body, mind, and spirit will help to balance your elements and the sacred geometry carried both within your cells and auric field. When you come together with your partner with the intention to create a child, the two of you will merge to create music. The combination of your love, chakras and energetic field matters.

Your child's sacred geometry and DNA will be affected by your vibration as a couple. The type of sound or frequency you are broadcasting will naturally create a specific type of child at conception. When you change the wavelength of your consciousness through the process of awakening, you will create a new frequency which is evidenced through your subtle vibrational quality. Everything in our world has a waveform creating unique patterns, signatures or sounds. When you and your partner come together to make love for the purpose of conception, it is vital that you be energetically aligned in order to create a third field of love.

Love sings a specific song matching that of Source. High-caliber souls will recognize their vibration within you.

At conception, the combined geometric fields of the couple will produce the base frequency of the baby. Yogi Bhajan taught that the sperm circles the egg exactly eight times and the force at which the sperm enters the egg creates the frequency of the child for the rest of their life. Higher dimensional fields carry subtle and specific energetic tones or sounds. In order to touch into these dimensional fields, for the purpose of conceiving a high-caliber child, you must carry a frequency which is similar to theirs. Dimensional fields are like octaves on the twelve-note scale. If your combined harmony matches these higher dimensional overtones, you will naturally conceive, hold, and birth light-filled children.

Unharmonious Relationships

Reaching these higher dimensional fields all sounds lovely until real life issues from earth come crashing down. Before I discuss how to create a higher frequency with your partner, I want to cover all of the behaviors that can sabotage your relationship so that you can become aware of them and take the steps needed to heal. A majority of relationships are ungrounded and cannot maintain trust, love, harmony, family dynamics, career changes, travel or fidelity. All of these issues need to be discussed and worked out in the process of becoming pregnant because they can create disease and disharmony, making conscious conception difficult. The everyday struggles of life create so many battles that the push and pull can exhaust us. I can teach you all about the energetics of creating a powerful soul, but if you aren't in alignment with your partner, there are bound to be issues that arise that may affect your fertility as a couple.

The benefit of negativity in relationships is that the feeling provides a place to expand from—a point of reference of what we do not want or need so that we can experience what we do want. Conscious conception requires couples to sit down together in order to plan having a baby and all the details that this includes. Intentional conversations bring clarity and balance. Before you have each baby, you must check in with your partner around critical life issues such as sex, finances, future goals, level of communication, and intimacy. Coming to a place of equanimity and synergy together as a couple will enhance the process of becoming pregnant and bring a great deal of harmony and respect into the relationship.

There are many personality flaws or ego mechanisms that can exist within relationships that create discordance between energy fields. When these types of underlying issues exist, you and your partner will not be able to create the high-frequency vibration or potent energetic third field of the Trinity. Unconditional love is something that humans usually touch into only for seconds, because our egos or personalities arise to create separation through our thought projections. Underneath the mind games is presence, which requires nothing from the other. Here are just a few examples of behaviors that can come between you and your partner which naturally create discordance in your fields.

Controlling or Domineering Behavior: Needing another person to act in a way that pleases you or meets your personal expectations of the world will naturally create a split. No one has the right to dictate rules or obligations to another on how to live their life. If they do so, it stems from a place of insecurity or even past trauma. This type of behavior can be seen in subtle ways, such as comments around what the other is wearing or how they look. Issues around freedom, what the other does with their spare time and who they spend their time with may arise. When someone experiences controlling behavior from another, it could potentially lower that individual's self-esteem, causing feelings of unworthiness and confusion. Boundaries need to be set and the relationship may require outside support.

Manipulation: This is experienced through subtle or obvious behaviors in words or actions. Manipulation often comes in the form of lengthy discourses or even an energy exchange that creates a power struggle. When someone begins to talk you out of your intuition or gut feeling about a behavior or situation, you need to take space to re-evaluate. The person may make you feel like you need them for happiness or survival. Using guilt tactics, which create shame, is not unusual. If someone is manipulating your energy, you may feel on edge, or energetically imbalanced around them. Healing requires an energetic balance in your relationship to bring peace. In order to dissolve the entanglement, it is necessary to work on issues around control and self-love.

Being Judgmental or Intolerant: This arises from personal insecurities that others mirror back to you about yourself. Judgment is a fast reaction to what we don't like about another or ourselves. It is a reference for our subconscious or personal projections. It is hard not to judge someone because our egos create a natural separation between bodies. The most important thing to do is learn how to catch yourself before you speak or act unkindly. Utilizing a group of friends to talk about your relationship issues is not a bad thing—women need to share issues in order to not place these problems on their partner.

Lack of Intimacy: I have had the great honor to work with many women in their process of becoming pregnant, and through our sessions it appears that couples have very similar relationship problems, especially when it comes to becoming pregnant. Those who struggle with fertility tend to lose deep intimacy because they are focused on the end result. The process of procreating becomes a marathon, rather than a unique and heightened experience—and that creates frustration. Intimacy comes in the form of conversation, touch, thoughtfulness, listening, holding one another and making love. When you are trying to become pregnant, all of these intimate behaviors should be at the forefront of your relationship to create a loving journey together.

Not Taking Responsibility for Actions: Avoiding personal faults and not owning your own issues will create massive separation in your relationship. If you are insecure, unhappy or angry, take the necessary steps to own your personal behavior. Say you are sorry when you are rude or short-tempered, especially if you expect the same from your partner. The projection that someone else is in the wrong is not worth your personal loss of energy. When you begin to take responsibility for your behavior, self-awareness grows. This will create a mirror for your partner to do the same.

Anger, Resentment, or Aggression: Keep in mind that anger is a mask for grief, sadness or fear. Do a personal inventory of the actions that create negative interactions within your relationship. Determine which emotions are driving your angry reactions. There is a three-minute Kundalini meditation, as taught by Yogi Bhajan, called Fists of Anger, which can be found with a quick Internet search. This meditation can be done more than once throughout the day and is excellent for reducing anger and aggression.

Lack of Communication: Conscious conversations require a balance of talking and listening. Scheduling in times to speak may not be a bad idea to ensure that conversations happen in a peaceful manner rather than an explosion of resentment. Communication is a critical component to a healthy relationship, but it requires vulnerability and honesty. It also works better if you are able to listen (and not think of what you are going to say next) while your partner is speaking. If your partner is struggling, sometimes all they want to hear is that you are there for them. The best ways to "fix" a situation may come through pure presence. When you speak with another, try to listen to the words that come out of your mouth. This active listening to yourself will bring greater awareness of whether your words are true, necessary, and coming from a space of love.

Projection: Catch yourself when you begin to project your subconscious trauma or neurosis onto your partner. According to Yogi Bhajan, women have eleven moon centers and men have only one. He said that the women who understand their moon centers will control this coming golden age. These moon centers fluctuate women's emotions every 2.5 days. Men don't have this type of fluctuation in moods as their energy stays grounded in their chin. Through self-work, I have become aware of my constant fluctuating moods as a result of the energetic shifts in my moon centers. Certain moon centers make women feel insecure, focused, flirty or even timid. If you get in tune with these shifts in mood, you can have more control of your behaviors and know where you will energetically be next. Understanding yourself brings greater clarity to your projections. Your only responsibility is to own your own behavior—and once you do this, you can lift the entire relationship.

Experiencing Guilt or Shame: Guilt is placed upon you by others. It makes you feel stuck because it stems from past experiences that are not actually happening in the present moment. When you absorb someone else's expectations of who you should be, you may be in a toxic situation. Guilt serves no purpose other than pulling negativity into a person's life—creating a darkness so that one cannot see clearly. Shame on the other hand holds the purpose of showing where improvements could take place. It occurs when you have contradicted your own morals. If you did all the right actions in a situation to the best of your ability, you need to let go of someone else's expectations of who you should be. If you didn't properly step up in a situation, learn from that, but do not dwell on it.

Relationships provide a catalyst for alchemical physical, spiritual, and emotional changes. When two highly connected souls meet traumas, unhealed wounds and subconscious patterns may arise for release. This provides the opportunity for internal growth and expansion. Once deep-rooted issues are worked through, the couple has the possibility of raising their frequency to a level of harmonic convergence with Source. If the two are meant to be together, and both have done their personal work, then their frequencies will unite as one. If one individual cannot keep up with the other person's level of growth, the Universe will likely provide the right partner for each to continually grow with the purpose of creating increased light within. The creation of love and harmony within the relationship is a critical component to the union and conscious conception.

Templates for a Sacred Marriage

There are templates of sacred marriage throughout history that provide some perspective of what a divine union looks like. These archetypes have set the stage for the conscious relationships that are beginning to form on Earth as the energetic frequency continues to rise. In the creation of the sacred marriage, the Holy Trinity is produced through three principles: the holy mother, the holy father and their divine child made of Spirit. Within a sacred relationship, there is a profound amount of energy between the male and female, which creates a third unified field. This field, which is often referred to as The Horus, can be amplified through sexual tantric practice. The couple will experience heightened consciousness because their chakras align, allowing the balanced energy of vulnerability and unconditional love to flow between them.

The first historical example of sacred marriage I will describe is that of the Queen of Sheba and King Solomon. As a high priestess, the Queen of Sheba understood the ritual of Hieros Gamos and was able to spend a period of time with her counterpart Solomon before they had to depart to separate lands. The Hieros Gamos is an ancient rite of passage in the holy marriage where two individuals make love on the physical plane and higher dimensional fields at the same time. It is an experience where the souls of the individuals, or their etheric light bodies, combine to create a heightened energy within and around them. The etheric light body was referred to as the Ka body, or etheric double, by the ancient Egyptians. The rite of passage was also an integral part of conceiving divine children in the ancient birthing temples of Greece. When Hieros Gamos takes place between a man and a woman, they are literally making love within a field of light. The experience feels like touching God through all of the senses. A somewhat similar experience can be created through tantric sexual practice.

The creation of light during sexual intercourse is a critical component of the creation of a holy child. The ancient art of creating light during sex is a tantric practice performed between a man and woman during lovemaking. Enlightened sexual encounters are not the average experience for most couples, but it sets a template of what is possible for you and your partner if you work to come together into higher union together. Though the Queen of Sheba and King Solomon's love encounter did not produce a child, it created a force of energy strong enough for Solomon to move forward with his destiny. He wrote a famous poem to honor his love called the Song of Solomon.

The second historical example is the twin soul union of the Goddess Isis and her male counterpart the God Osiris, which created the nation of Egypt and made a lasting impact on history. Their combined energy created their son Horus, a powerful leader and also a worshipped God known for his light. Another example, and one I have already discussed, is the union between the divine couple Mary Magdalene and Jesus, which has been hidden throughout history. Through their sacred union, and the practice of the Hieros Gamos, Mary helped Jesus to prepare for resurrection (as Isis did for Osiris). Though historical texts do not publish this, Mary Magdalene also birthed Jesus' child. If you want to learn more about this, I encourage you to research the Gospel of Mary Magdalene and read *The Magdalene Manuscript* by Tom Kenyon. This text describes the Hieros Gamos and tantric union in detail. This alchemical sexual union can be practiced between you and your partner to help you reach higher levels of love for the purpose of conscious conception.

These couples all held deep devotion to their Source and completion within themselves. When the polarity of the male and female came together in this wholeness, a lasting legacy of unconditional love was created which altered history. A woman in alignment with her true nature will always be creating. Her creations will either be constructive or destructive, depending on her level of consciousness. If a woman is not creating a book, business, poetry or any actual physical manifestation, she can transfer that energy to creating a child. Within the relationship of a divine union, her power to create is amplified because of the level of support and reverence that she feels from her counterpart. When a woman feels deep trust, love, and intimacy from her partner at conception and during pregnancy, these emotions will dramatically affect the environment of their growing child and his/her DNA.

Connecting with Your Beloved for Conscious Conception

Sexual intercourse performed for the purpose of conscious conception is a chemical romance and alchemical union between the male and female. When a couple is in balance, they have complementary sacred geometry within their energetic fields. This creates a unique vibration between all of their chakras and increased alignment. Their combined love forms a palpable physical energy which is amplified during sexual intercourse. Senses become heightened and conscious awareness increases. As we know from the beginning of the book, the senses play a key role in forming the energetic signature and sacred geometry of the child at conception.

Ensuring that you and your partner are free from domestic issues, and fully aligned in your bodies, minds, and spirits will not only enhance your fertility, but the type of soul you will birth. Conception should ideally be a planned event where the two of you speak about bringing a child into the world before you find out you are pregnant. I went into great detail about this in *Mystical Motherhood*. The book includes information on important concepts to discuss with your partner and how to amplify your fields in the seventy-two hours before conception. In *Fertile*, I want you to leave with a deeper understanding about what a divine relationship looks like and what it does not. Many relationships are caught in negative repeating patterns which block the mind, heart, and sacral region from connecting—and connection is vital to conscious conception.

The aligning of your energy fields creates a direct conduit to the higher dimensions or planes of existence where your child is waiting with a matching frequency. Your chakras are similar to a piano keyboard with various notes that hit different harmonics. They create their own unique sounds, colors, and experiences of reality. If all the keys, or energetic centers, are aligned between the two of you during sexual intercourse, you will hit the highest octave. This sexual bliss creates specific geometry, music, and mathematics which imprint the cells of your egg.

Your harmony reverberates out and attracts the dimensional reality that it corresponds to. For example, if you and your partner are only aligned at the base chakra, and living in survival mode, you will create a vibration, sound, color, and geometry at the time of conception that will attract a child with a similar frequency. If you only have the three lower chakras in alignment, the two of you will emit a denser energetic signature. In order to create a holy child, the male and the female should ideally be aligned energetically at every chakra, creating a cosmic divine dance of bliss during sexual intercourse. The love created at conception produces a template and a blueprint of the DNA within the egg.

Sacred Sexuality and Creating the Third Unified Field with Your Partner

When a couple comes together as one to make love, two spherical fields are energetically formed creating the vesica piscis—the sacred geometrical figure presented in the Spirit chapter. The person simply becomes an extension of yourself and the other body can be considered your own. This feeling of oneness has no sound because it creates presence. It makes no requests and it requires no control. When thoughts are released and power struggles are non-existent, all rules, expected outcomes, pressure, and force are eliminated. Enlightened sex creates union.

Sacred love is an energetic connection that creates pure reverence for the other. Thoughts of who is wrong or right are dropped. The most important question is "How can I serve you so that I in turn serve myself?" The creation of this unification allows the Holy Spirit to recognize itself through the combination of your energies. When you are in a holy union, you have found the Beloved here on Earth. As the two spherical auric fields come together, they will create a unified third field. This energy can be transferred into the creation of a child.

You will know that the third field is formed when a heightened level of intimacy, trust, love, and compassion dances between the two of you. This energy may feel like a chemical drug, yet it does not dissipate. It is a palpable force that creates tantric energy between a couple both while apart and in each other's company. On a visceral level, every cell has come alive. In this type of relationship, both the masculine and the feminine are fully healed and whole within themselves. They do not come together to work out their old wounds or patterns for clearing, because if they did, the third field would not form or hold within these lower vibrations. They unite because they chose one another, and they know that their choice to bring down a holy child is an act of worship for one another and the Universe.

In this third field, unique relationship, the intellect is stimulated through conversation, the heart is expanded through mutual respect and the sacral regions of the two are highly engaged even when physically separated. When the two come together in conscious sexual intercourse, they form a chalice and also have the ability to create a significant amount of light. The creation of this light can be practiced by focusing on the eighth chakra, or Ka body, at the time of orgasm and expanding outward. Again, I refer you to Tom Kenyon's *The Magdalene Manuscript* should you want to explore this more deeply.

Your Journey to Union

A FEW QUESTIONS TO REFLECT UPON:

- *What wounds or patterns remain unhealed between you and your partner? Do you have a plan to work through these or resources to help?*

- *Where do you place blame or not take responsibility for your own actions?*

- *Do you feel comfortable accepting love? How do you or your partner push love away?*

- *In what ways do you become rigid or shut down sexually, emotionally, or physically with your partner? Why do you do this? Can you open more?*

- *When you really want something from your partner, such as touch, have you ever practiced giving it first?*

- *How can you increase intimacy through touch, praise, serving, and loving your partner?*

- *How do you communicate—and are the methods that you are using effective?*

SPIRIT — THE CIRCLE

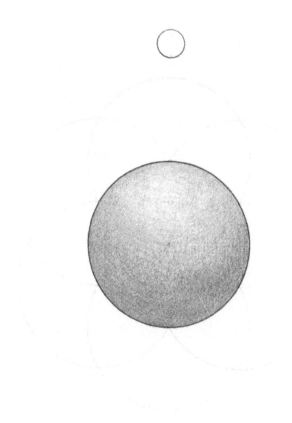

sphere

CHAPTER 7

ALCHEMICAL TRANSFORMATION AND
THE POWER OF THE ELEMENTS

Imagine a monad, or single cell, at the time of conception glowing like the sun within your womb, ripe with the energy of creation. As the programming of this singular entity begins, Spirit pours in from every angle forming a blueprint of consciousness. Light intermixes with sound to form the base elements of your child. Sacred geometry, your six senses, your level of awareness and the universal elements are all involved in the process of creation. If your elements are balanced at the time of conception, the baby's blueprint will form in a neutral and calm environment. This is not always the circumstance and an imbalance of fire, water, air, earth or ether can cause emotional, mental, and physical unease.

The Universe is made up of 108 elements, but you only have to focus on the five I have already discussed with you for the purpose of conscious conception. In chapter four I discussed how the elements internally affect your body and alter your life. Now I would like you to understand how the elements can affect you from the outside world.

Spirit utilizes the elements to help you through the process of awakening, causing internal alchemical transformation. When you are going through a period of change, it is good to know which element is affecting your life so that you can counterbalance the energy. This is especially important when you are trying to become pregnant, because the elements are connected to the sacred geometry that programs your child. They help to create an energetic signature and architectural composition at conception and throughout gestation. Creating an internal balance, even when you are going through a spiritual awakening, can help to form a centered child.

If you are reading this book, you are reaching for a higher level of self-awareness and are on the path of awakening to your divinity. You may be going through a transformative process and I don't want you to feel alone in your journey. When I was going through my personal spiritual awakening, I wish I had had a better understanding of just how much the elements were alchemically changing my life. It would have helped me to get a grip on a situation that often felt out of control. When you feel the effects of outside forces or pressure that makes you change, this is God and your Higher Self working to accelerate you. Spirit applies alchemy to your life to help you grow, and in the spiral of becoming, your consciousness will constantly be refined through the power of fire, water, air, earth, and ether.

The Transformative Power of Alchemy

Fire: The first step of the alchemical transformation is calcination which, as I discussed earlier, corresponds to the element of fire in your life. Calcination reduces everything to ashes and psychologically burns off the density of your personality and belief systems. When the element fire begins to affect your world, you will lose attachments to the material realm and free yourself from your own self-deception. Fire vigorously works on the ego and mind. The separation from a false reality and our attachments can be a painful process to go through.

Water: The element water creates the process of dissolution within your life. It helps us let go of relationships and paths not meant for us. Water cleanses and dissolves structures to create new patterns. This receptive element also helps to form your intuition and psychic abilities. This part of the spiritual transformation will take you to the watery depths of despair and provides a better understanding of all of your unresolved emotions. As you release all that does not serve you, you will be baptized and reborn.

Air: The element air is like the breath of God coming to carry you where you are supposed to be in life. The wind element can produce dramatic, unpredictable or sudden changes in your environment. Air is a life force which helps to move you out of stagnancy. Anytime that you are resistant to change, the element air will swiftly move through to amplify your emotions around what is holding you back. Air helps to create separation from old habits or ways of being. The element makes decisive splits and life-changing decisions possible.

Earth: The earth element is related to conjunction, which is the process of coming together, of unification and the full embodiment of spirit within your human form. When this element is active in your life, there will be a coming to-gether of the creative and receptive forces. It is the union within of the male and female, yin and yang, and sun and moon. At this stage of spiritual transformation, you may encounter people who are your opposite energetically. These individ-uals will help you to look at life differently. By experiencing opposing forces, you become grounded and in union within. Earth helps to ground and embody both your spiritual process and all of the energetic changes that you have gone through so far in your awakening.

Ether: Ether uses a higher alchemical process to help you move from an earthly, or three-dimensional, level of understanding into the heavenly realms, or higher planes of existence. It opens up the mystical, mysterious, and esoter-ic secrets of the Universe. When you are in this level of transformation, your imagination becomes your greatest tool as duality dissolves. You will find that there is no such thing as above or below—it all becomes One. By this point in the alchemical transformation, you are highly connected to the divine and have surrendered yourself to Spirit. You know that nothing is under your control. A higher consciousness becomes the primary director of your life. In this phase, you have moved from density to the subtle realms of existence and become light.

Determining your level of inner alchemy, and what elements are affecting your life, can be done by paying attention to what is happening in your environment and how you react to it. The elements that are primarily running your energy at the time of conception will significantly program your baby because they have an environmental impact on your level of consciousness. If you can identify what is happening on the inside, and how it correlates to what is occurring in your outside world, you will have an easier time identifying the level of alchemical transformation that you are going through.

Remember that genes are programmed by environmental input. If you conceive your baby at a time when you are, for example, primarily experiencing the element of fire, and your consciousness is being transformed, your child's basic characteristics will be significantly affected by this element. Identifying a particular element early on will allow you to compensate by using other elements energetically and physically throughout the rest of your pregnancy, with the intention of balancing out the makeup of your child's energetic composition. The goal is to create harmony in the sacred geometrical human design and resemble nature in a balanced state.

My Spiritual Transformation and Journey Through the Elements

The first time I realized that the elements are a part of our internal and external spiritual journey was in a Vipassana meditation center in the woods in northern California. It was created by a man from India, S.N. Goenka, who opened spiritual centers across the world for the purpose of holding three and ten-day silent meditation courses. I could not look at another person, read, exercise or use the Internet for ten days. The silence was torturous, but I did learn a lot about myself. The experience helped me to realize that each of the elements discussed here can be felt pulsating through our bodies.

These elements represent our karmas, past lives and DNA templates, which can all be found within the structures of our muscles, organs, and bones. As I sat in that communal room hour after hour, I could feel the density in my cells weighing me down. Thoughts felt like the wind blowing vigorously. Physical pain would arise like fire, burning in my muscles. Water would move through me, creating either waves of emotion or moments of relief. I witnessed my resistances and watched them dissipate. The silence taught me that we are primarily composed of elements and can internally adjust them through our spiritual practice.

As mentioned previously, my spiritual journey began as a rollercoaster after a spontaneous Kundalini awakening, which felt like the Universe running through my spine and consciousness with a tremendous amount of strength. This energy forces you to find God in all forms so that you can eventually find the Beloved within. An outside force is usually required to make us find ourselves and connect back to Spirit. Your transformational journey may have begun through infertility. Sickness, death, birth or major changes can also make us reevaluate our lives. These outside forces help us to look in the mirror and process our past, so that we can move towards our destiny, which usually has something to do with healing our biggest wounds so that we can teach others what we have learned.

My alchemical transformation felt similar to psychological and physical surgery as I was forced to look at all the ways I attempted to find happiness, love, and Source outside of myself. This process shifted my belief systems, familial or earthly bonds, relationships, and career. My consciousness was redesigned and my DNA changed. Spirit helped me find self-mastery and internal power by applying outside pressure through the energetic effects of the elements. When you begin to awaken, there is a general pattern that is helpful to understand as fire, water, air, earth, and ether move through your life creating changes. Just when you think you have cleared yourself, another level of up-leveling occurs and the alchemical process repeats itself.

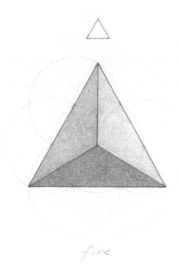

fire

Fire: The Triangle or Tetrahedron

The element fire is a catalyst for your greatest expansion. It is the first element used in ancient alchemy by Spirit for the purpose of awakening. The heat it creates burns you up to clean you out, forcing deep pain to arise for the purpose of elimination. Fire tends to destroy everything in its path when it is not contained internally or externally. If you are experiencing the fire element in events outside of yourself, it will usually come in the form of what may feel like a combustible cosmic explosion. Anything that causes you to suddenly wake up and take a look at the way you are living your life is fire in action.

The experience of fire is painful and it moves fast and furiously to create change. An intense fight or affair could ruin a relationship. A chance meeting may ignite something in you that could alter your life forever. A divorce, passionate love affair, revolution or explosive fight are all examples of the power of fire in the outward world. Your soul aligns with Spirit to create these events so that you can excel. The friction of the experience forces you to change and often move faster than your personality is ready to. This is all part of the deconstruction of your ego. Emotions such as passion, anger, frustration, rage, and a need for control or power arise in order to be faced and eliminated.

Fire brings rapid changes that we can either resist or surrender to. It heats you up until your world turns to ashes by creating massive shifts of perception that humble you to a higher force. The element takes away our material attachments. Anything that you think you need for survival or that you cling to cannot stand the flames. This may be a relationship, house, way of being or possessions. We think we are in control and it requires a large combustion to show us that we are not. Fire helps to remove the barriers in your life, shakes your view of reality, and redefines who you are. This type of shift creates a great deal of introspection and self-evaluation because you will finally be able to experience yourself without the person, place or thing that was holding you back.

I personally spent five years with the element fire and watched it burn away my job, specific friends, and my way of interacting with the world. I also became pregnant with both of my children while the fire element was altering my life. I birthed two very intense and spirited souls as a result. At the time, I did not know about the concepts I am teaching you now, because they were not at my level of consciousness. Looking back, I wish I had been more aware of my internal response to the life changes I was going through and used other elements to counterbalance the heat. It is important to know what element is working on your life when you become pregnant so that you understand what is environmentally affecting your child. There is nothing wrong with being programmed primarily by one element, but you should at least be aware of what is happening to you spiritually so that you can consciously decide to balance out your internal response or not.

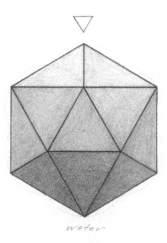

water

Water: The Icosahedron

After the element fire moved vigorously through my life, I felt the cooling presence of water flow through and dissolve what was left of the ashes. The element brought relief, but also its own unique set of challenges. Water allows a period of looking inward and reflecting upon what the fire element burned away. Lunar energies become heightened. Feeling, intuition, and emotion are magnified as Spirit enters to resurrect you into a new life. The cleansing and baptizing effect helps you to truly let go of what no longer serves your higher purpose. The element asks, "Are you now open and willing to become fluid in order to alter your life?"

Water creates change by intensifying emotions. Numbness does not connect us to God—feelings do. We don't have to ruminate on our emotions, but we must express them. This is a critical part of the process of awakening because it brings you back to life. Once you feel the sadness, depression, doubt, fear, and resistances, your senses will awaken. The world becomes vivid in touch, sound, taste, and pulsating energy. Suppression of emotion creates layer after layer of density which makes our souls expressionless within our bodies. Emotions such as sadness or grief may arise as you come to realize that certain friends might not be genuine, that family members are toxic or the love of your life is not the right person for you. Discovering these truths can be painful, but the dissolving of these situations allows a fresh outlook and more space for new experiences.

Water helps you to fully let go of situations that you have been holding onto for many years or even lifetimes. Whatever is blocking you from expanding into divinity, or keeping you trapped in the human story of drama and trauma, must release. Water is destabilizing, as it requires that you dissolve your rigidity and need for control. It assists in purifying the ego so that fewer judgments are present and more truth can flow through without the preconceptions of the personality. You may need to take time to be alone for self-reflection and solitude in order for all of these changes to take place.

Being alone creates a period of regeneration. The moon, which is connected to water, disappears in the night sky throughout the month. When you are spiritually experiencing this element, you may need to disappear too. Time spent in solitude and silence is necessary—it helps you to connect to your Higher Self and soul. You will learn to listen to God rather than the outside world for guidance. A common theme in the process of awakening is a period of feeling extreme isolation. Know that you are not alone and ask for help if the depression or intense emotions do not lift. During this time, you are submerging yourself into your subconscious and the center of your being. This period lifts the constraints and attachments of the outside world and reveals who you truly are. Rather than looking outward for love and belonging, you find this experience within.

I have gone through many periods in my life where I felt completely alone in my process of awakening. This feeling of loneliness helped me to realize that I was never actually by myself and that Source was always with me. When I spent time in reflection, I began to see God in everything. Leaves that fell from the trees appeared as sacred. The songs on the radio sounded like they were messages sent just for me. The conversations I had with random individuals provided the answers to my prayers. The element water helped to purify my mind so that I could see that I was the creator of my own reality. I recognized that my thoughts and feelings dictated what occurred in my world.

Water will enhance your psychic or clairvoyant sensitivities so that you can fully connect to Source. Riding the waves, which may oscillate between elation and depression, is necessary in order to find clarity within your center. You will learn to trust yourself. Signs will appear as guideposts. The synchronicities that happen to you will no longer be considered random. Once you dissolve within, you also dissolve into God. As everything becomes One, Spirit will begin to whisper into your ear as the cosmic breath of God flows through you. This breath is the element of air, which is the next alchemical step in your transformational journey. Wind will move you where you need to go next in life.

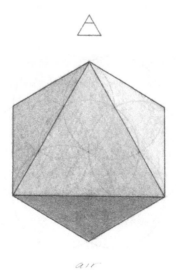

air

Air: The Octahedron

When you are stagnant or spiritually resistant to change, you can be sure that wind will enter your life to create upheaval. Air tells you where to go and how to get there. It is an uplifting element that will take you from living a mediocre life to experiencing a world like no other. An existence full of surprises and growth. The element air makes individuals move beyond their comfort zones and usually at a more rapid rate than normal because it alchemizes ordinary reality into cosmic consciousness. Air confronts day-to-day life and creates a different world view.

When the element air entered my life, I began a wild dragon ride. After a period of dissolution, where I spent a couple of years processing all the changes I was going through spiritually, wind came to carry me away. I moved to Europe and left my reality as I knew it. My life at the time looked mundane, yet perfect from the outside. I lived in a wealthy community with trees, trails, good schools, expensive grocery stores, and smiling people. I thought that success looked a certain way and contained a certain number of items, resources, and relationships. This reality does not equate to success for everyone, though that is what society would like us to believe.

After moving to Europe, I learned what prosperity truly means. A massive amount of traveling helped me to redefine what success is for me personally. My journey to living an abundant life was also a journey of self-creation. I traveled the world for two years, visiting sacred sites across five continents and around twenty countries. These experiences activated various memories in me of my soul's purpose and provided the material for *Mystical Motherhood* and this book. Wind helped to unravel whatever was left of my need for control. It released all the ways that I had once imprisoned myself through material belongings, houses, career, concept of self or environment. I lost self-importance as I realized just how big the world is and how powerful Spirit can be when you surrender. Following that clear voice inside leads you to where you are supposed to go next. Even if you have no plan, it is your eternal yes to life.

Air helps you become comfortable with the unpredictable. It provides whispers from God, which guide you to make necessary changes in your life in order to meet the people you need to, or go to the places that will change your destiny. Commit to the journey, not the destination. The element can help you let go of society's expectations of what life looks like around money, home, and relationships. Your journey is personal, and only you can define what success and growth look like. Spiritual transformation creates the masterpiece of your life.

If you are feeling imprisoned by old habits or ways of being, do not be surprised if wind comes in to redirect you on your path. Invoke this element to help you break away. Even if you think your life is perfect, I promise you it can get better and the only thing holding you back is your fear of change. This is your biggest obstacle to spiritual growth—love doesn't live where fear thrives. Air helps your consciousness to expand internally and externally. It lifts you into Heaven and creates a deeper trust and communication with Source. Once you feel the exhilarating effects of flying free in the higher realms, you will have to take what you learned from wind and apply it back to your daily life. This is the meaning of true embodiment. As you ground spiritual success into the everyday world, you begin to work with the element of earth.

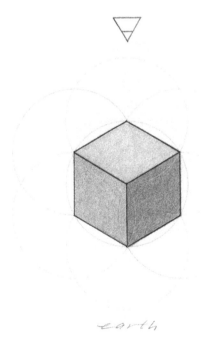

earth

Earth: The Cube or Hexahedron

Earth is the representation of solid matter. It is the creation and embodiment of Spirit in action. The element earth puts the divine spark of God within man in order to go out into the world and solidify higher spiritual principles into everyday life. Once the creative and receptive parts of you have come together, the earth element will enter your life to create internal union. This union is formed when the male and female principle parts have come together in a sacred marriage within. When this occurs, there is less looking outside of yourself for happiness because you have solidified with the divine in your human form. This embodiment creates alignment between Heaven and Earth so that you can complete what you came here to do.

It is just as important to ground into the earth as it is to reach up for the stars. After traveling the world, I knew it was time to build a permanent home so that I could create more books for you to consume. I had to embody the spiritual principles I had learned through my alchemical transformation over a seven-year time span. As the earth element spiritually moved through me, I began to see all the ways that the constant movement of the wind created distraction and anxiety in my mind and body. Air is necessary to lift stagnancy in our lives, but it should not create a constant hurricane. When we come into internal balance, there is equanimity in being and doing. The earth element creates inner stillness and anchors you in your mission.

This embodiment of Spirit on Earth is the key to changing our planet and creating a higher frequency that expands for all to experience. For years, I felt anxiety because I knew I had come here to do something important. Every moment I was not completing my mission felt like a massive amount of time lost. An inner union of Heaven and Earth was required for me to truly produce in this realm. If you ever feel like you came here to do something, but you cannot remember what it is, the earth element can help you materialize it. Earth assists with creation.

We have lost our ability to tap into the energy of this planet and have forgotten to ask for help from our Mother Earth to materialize matter. If you want to create something, such as a baby, it is necessary to ground your energy down into the earth for stabilization. Earth will help you to become pregnant and safely hold the baby. An exercise I mentioned earlier: you can ground your energy by imagining roots that grow from your spine into the middle of the Earth. This will take away a lot of your anxiety and help you to release stress.

The element solidifies time and space, Heaven and Earth, and the ability to do and be. It can heal insecurity and the need for constant activity, which is another form of depression. Many people have the belief that one cannot be both financially success-ful and spiritual. When you are fully embodying your true nature, you should be able to hold both the material and spiritual realms with ease. Your manifestation abilities will become very powerful because you will know how to materialize. Embodiment of Spirit on Earth is the only way we can truly make things happen for the better and move on to completing our destiny.

The difference between fate and destiny is that fate is controlled by your subcon-scious programming and karma. Fate is similar to being bounced around like a soccer ball in life. It is not fun, especially if you are not consciously aware that you are even a part of a game. What you believe is your next step is actually just the past coming in to be cleared. When you begin to act upon your destiny on Earth, you have cleared much of your past programming and become consciously aware of every move. Life on Earth is surrendered to Spirit and resembles a game of chess, but you are now an expert player. When you become a master, you can see how each move will play out and know beforehand how to act in relationships and experiences. When you are living your destiny, you will make a global impact that creates a positive imprint for others to excel into their greatest selves. At this point you move into ether easily.

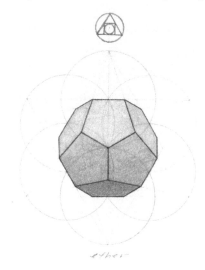

ether

Ether: The Circle or Pentagonal Dodecahedron

The element ether is your conscious connection to God, Spirit, Source, and light on Earth. The element teaches you that your most important relationship is the one you have with your own divinity. Cultivating this will allow you to create beyond what most human beings think is possible. Heal beyond what most people comprehend and teach beyond what most individuals can understand. Ether helps you touch into the Heavens in order to bring unknown knowledge back for others. It provides evolved humans with secrets that are generations ahead of their time because it sharpens the ability to listen and know the truth.

Ancient alchemists have a saying, "As above so below," which means having your feet consciously in both the material and spiritual worlds in order to co-create a new reality. Expansive experiences of the divine dissolve you into pure consciousness in order to remind you where you came from. The alchemical process described in this chapter will repeat itself until you are refined and clear enough to experience this level of reality. This requires constant letting go and surrendering—which also happen to be important qualities for fertility. When you begin to feel the element ether, you will experience God all around you. Your waking world will not just be the density of the three-dimensional, which you normally experience on Earth, because you will anchor a fifth-dimensional existence of higher vibrations. Ether invokes the high spiritual masters to assist you, especially in your process of becoming a mother.

The element enters our lives in profound ways. When individuals witness angels, saints or sages completing miracles through visitations, this is a gift from God. I personally experienced ether the night I was asked to write this book. A trusted teacher asked me over to her house on a full moon. We completed a ceremony, and as she held my hand in this world, my pineal gland opened up to higher dimensions, and I merged with my Higher Self. This gave me a three-hundred-sixty=degree view revealing the dimensional fields to my awareness. This divine intervention rewired my brain and allowed me to utilize my third eye, which created an expansive view of reality and a new frequency in my being. I gained the ability to see, hear, and feel fully. I visually saw and felt myself walking out of my body and into higher planes of existence where I was greeted by many

Ascended Masters. These masters have stayed with me; I created a lasting relationship with them and that has propelled me forward in life.

These experiences, and the ability to interact with the divine, will become common for individuals as we move into this enlightened age. This is your divine right and inheritance as a creator on Earth. These angelic guides are here to help, but you must ask for their assistance—they cannot intervene without your invitation. When ether enters your life, prayer, devotion, and meditation become an essential part of your day. This helps you surrender and allow Spirit to guide you into full alignment. It creates presence, and moment-by-moment trusting. The unknown becomes comfortable and the Universe provides all you need when you need it.

In order to see it, you have to believe it. To experience the saints, sages, and masters, you must begin to let go of your sense of entitlement and knowing. Your past belief systems of what is possible or impossible, right or wrong, must dissolve in order for you to merge with reality. Heaven exists on Earth and your density blocks you from experiencing this—as do many religious affiliations that claim that Source is found outside of you. Ether connects you to the process of ascension, which is the path of going home. As you feel your microcosmic Self merge with your macrocosmic existence while here on Earth, you are on the fast track to letting go of the human story and becoming a fully awakened human being.

'Christ' Means a Form That is Carrying Something Holy

If you are on the path of conceiving and birthing an enlightened or high-caliber child, you are going to go through a vast amount of spiritual changes. Your womb carries the energetic signature to creating a child unlike any other. Spiritual advancement is not just a choice—it is an absolute necessity for your state of consciousness and ability to complete this intention. Elements are the tools that Spirit uses to help you awaken to divinity and purify your vessel.

An alchemical process of transformation continually happens throughout life, whether you are aware of it or not. Once you experience the elements (which may take one year or ten) you will move through them all again and sometimes in tandem. In this chapter, I only covered the basic elemental principles to spiritual progression. Your own spiritual journey will be unique to you and reveal the process of becoming gold. As you rise like the phoenix from the ashes of what you once knew as life, you will be able to look back and have a clearer picture of just how much help you had from a higher power on your road to self-discovery.

The basic description provided here gives you a better understanding of the spiritual process of awakening so that you will be able to pinpoint what element is affecting you and choose your reaction to these outside circumstances. Trust me, this is a gift. I did not have this knowledge until many years into my spiritual journey. Most people who go through an awakening, or any amount of growth, have no idea what is going on and little guidance for how to handle it.

The word 'Christ' means a form that is carrying something holy. You are literally embodying Feminine Christ Consciousness for the planet in your process of becoming the best version of yourself. As you prepare your body, mind, and spirit for conscious conception and pregnancy, it is inevitable that you will transform into an entirely new human. This is because you are being prepared to birth and raise an entirely new type of energetic soul. The alchemical process is your guidepost as to how Spirit is helping you make these internal changes. In your journey to becoming the divine feminine archetype and Holy Chalice, a lot of issues will arise to be released.

Growth can feel never-ending and exhausting at times. You will be pushed to your limits in a constant state of contraction and then expansion of your soul's essence or Spirit. These experiences stretch the nervous system which cultivates a deep inner strength. The greater the expansion, the more energetic bandwidth you will be able to hold. Old relationships and patterns that once triggered you will fade from your consciousness as your auric field grows large enough to contain something holy: a sacred child. In order to feel this vibration, it is necessary to drop who you think you are supposed to be in order to become who you really are.

Spirit wants to recognize itself in you, and constant refinement is necessary to do so. When you become accustomed to what element is working within your life, you can choose to move through the changes with grace and less reaction. The purpose is to let go of all resistances. Surrendering to a higher force will ultimately bring you the freedom you have always wanted. You cannot control how Spirit, and your Higher Self, utilize the elements to help you grow. You can, however, identify what element is affecting you and determine if you are going to resist the changes or allow them to transform you. Reactions to life changes program your baby during pregnancy. Training yourself to hold a sense of stillness through spiritual alchemy will create a balanced soul.

Becoming the Cosmic Creatrix

There are some very unique places in the world which actively use the elements in ceremony, thus creating a high vibration and connection to Spirit within the land. Bali and a few locations in India come to mind, as these cultures maintain active spiritual practices which help to activate the environments, living spaces, and temples. The communities of these locations hold deep devotion to Source and place importance upon creating ritual, utilizing the elements as a part of their daily practice or way of living. Ritual creates a palpable feeling of peace and expansion within the person and the surrounding area. In Bali, I could feel Spirit pulsating through the land because of the level of love that the Balinese have for their Hindu Gods. Their meditation practice and devotion to keeping active altars create a feeling of aliveness within every cell.

Devotion to the Creator through active ritual, dance, or singing is something that Western culture significantly lacks. There is weakness in our spirits and we ooze neurotic tendencies to control time, work, love, and people. We spend most of our lives indoors using light switches rather than starting a fire. We have lost our connection to the elements and do not honor their power. As a result, we are not even aware that they are our lifelines back to God. The Spirit world is here to assist us in our process of remembering who we are. Becoming cognizant of the elements within and without will help you to recreate this connection and pulsate as one with the Universe.

If you want to become the Holy Chalice, it is not only important to take the necessary steps and initiations to come into union with your Higher Self, but you also need to create devotion to Source. When ceremonies or rituals are carried out, they usually use the elements to invoke a higher power. Making your home into an active temple with an altar is not just for spiritual materialism or show—it is an absolute necessity. If your environment is vibrating from the love and devotion you have put into this, your cells will respond. An altar is the representation of your internal spiritual growth and devotion to Source. Sacred spaces should be formed to honor losses, joys, changes, people, places, deaths, prayers, or love. Revering your inner process in an outward way will help you to process and transform.

Create an altar that holds all of the elements in some form that is special to you. You can gather pieces of wood, stones, crystals, leaves, feathers or specific colored candles. Your altar can also contain photos, sacred objects or statues. Create a space to represent your journey to fertility and all the progress you have made. It should only hold objects of spiritual significance and should not be touched by others unless you are comfortable with that.

If you are being affected by a certain element, honor that change in your sacred space. Counterbalancing the effects of elements in an outward way will help your consciousness navigate internally. An example of this would be including extra water on the altar if you are dealing with fire in your life. You can also use the space to invoke the elements for support, manifestation, changes or balance. Pray and meditate within your sacred space or create multiple areas in your home which hold this type of energy. Everyone who enters your home will naturally feel the spiritual essence of the heightened environment, and as a result your awakening will touch them too.

Utilizing the Elements on Your Own Spiritual Journey

You can utilize the elements in your own spiritual practice for alchemical transformation just using your imagination and prayers. Here are a few examples of how to do this:

+ When I am working with a client who has a repeating pattern, I help her to remember the times in her life where she felt the emotion before. We energetically gather all of the memories that are hiding somewhere in her bones, tissues, organs or energetic centers and collect them into an imaginary container. I ask my client to visually see and feel these memories before energetically removing them. We use fire to burn these memories from her consciousness, water to cleanse and put out the fire, wind to blow the water away and earth to soak up whatever is left of the memories. A similar meditation was provided to you at the beginning of this book.

✤ If you are having a repeated problem at work with a coworker who is perhaps bullying you, a good way to handle this type of outside fire element is to become consciously aware that this person is not your enemy, but an angel. Someone who has come into your life to help you heal a deep wound. When he or she comes into your field and begins to trigger you, become aware of other times this has happened: perhaps with your mother, father or siblings. Find any specific memories linked to this same feeling or situation. Go through each memory one by one and place them in a glass jar in your mind's eye. Then imagine the elements as described above energetically moving the memories out of your body.

✤ The elements can be invoked to create balance and change. In order to govern these elements, you must embrace them, because you cannot truly have a relationship to anything that you aren't connected to. If you are feeling stuck or cannot make a decision, call upon the element of air for assistance. If you need to let go of a person in your life, utilize the element water. Place blessed bowls of water around your home, go swimming or shower. Utilize fire to burn away old patterns, memories, trauma or pain. Call upon earth to ground you or to build a stronger foundation in your home or work life. Invoke ether by calling upon the angels, saints, and sages for assistance.

✤ If you are being assailed by fire and feel that everything is up in flames around you, which is causing you to literally lose your grip on reality, become comfortable with the element. Burn candles, light fires in your fireplace, utilize the element in ceremony to burn letters or for meditation. You can do this with each of the elements individually by keeping an active altar which honors your spiritual progression and dreams of creating a family.

CHAPTER 8

INVOKING THE EIGHT
ASPECTS OF SELF

The ancient Hermetic or alchemist principle of "as above so below" also means "as within so without." Throughout the book I have discussed how the environment, experienced through your six senses, affects your internal self. In chapter seven, I also went into great detail on how Spirit can energetically affect you internally via outside influences through the process of alchemical transformation. Now I want you to fully understand the internal experience of God rushing through you, affecting your surrounding environment and touching every person and place you come in contact with. When Spirit runs through you like this, you will fully understand what God is and embody the Beloved on Earth.

A fully awakened human being vibrates at a unique frequency and reverberates the Beloved from within. They are fully alive, pulsating with energy which can be physically felt and visually seen through their eyes. Many people vibrate this continuously, but the majority of individuals on the planet yearn to experience this feeling even just once in their lifetime. This vibration is similar to the way that nature thrives. Lush with fertility and pregnant with life, Mother Earth lives to produce beauty. She thrives by serving others with her energy. The true nature of life is that we live in an ocean of love. When we relax and feel safe, this energy pours forth. When the Beloved flows through your physical body and soul you will feel this love, abundance, and happiness in full expansion. This vibration is unlike any other feeling on the planet because it is Source or God rushing through you. It heals and offers energy like light from the sun.

The vibration is not only nourishing to your soul, but it replenishes those around you. An individual emitting this frequency becomes a full vessel, over-flowing with the greater aspects of the Universe. Higher thoughts of unity, trust, union, respect, harmony, truth, and reverence for all pour out in order to serve others for the highest good. Most people constantly chase this experience outside of themselves, as they believe that relationships, money, sex, drugs or food will lead to this type of happiness. Yet, these outside influences can't sustain a high vibration and will quickly fade like the effects of a drug do. Once you cultivate the Beloved inside yourself, you will truly understand that nothing else can make you happier than vibrating the cosmos.

When the Beloved starts to flow through, you become a walking Goddess on Earth. Plants glow, the birds sound sweeter and food tastes better. Life may ap-pear a little softer sensually, and visually you may even see a soft glow. As your consciousness expands, you begin to pay attention to just how perfect it all is. You will see Source in everything and everyone. People in turn will experience the Beloved mirrored back to them through you. This is a blessing, but can some-times cause trouble. When an ocean of love is emitted through one person's heart center and experienced by another, it is frequently misinterpreted as romantic—when it is not. Rather than seeing the love for what it is, which is the essence of being on a quantum level, people tend to individuate and divide spiritual experi-ences into people, places or even things. This is the nature of humanity, but it is a quality that can easily change when you create a balanced elemental state within.

Love can be experienced at this molecular level only when vulnerability and openness to receive is flowing. Your energy must be non-threatening in order to emit the frequency of the Beloved. There can be no fear in any form. The energy holds no judgments, no urge to control, no jealousy, envy or pride. Perception by the senses cannot be the dominant force when this type of vibration is run-ning through you. This is because smells, visual effects and sounds often create memories to past experiences, which take you out of the present moment. When this happens, your mind judges the other person based on false belief systems.

You must experience others through your subtle essence and allow thoughts and words to become connected with the higher realms. There should be no identification involved. The other person will in turn experience the way that you feel as you are experiencing them. When someone feels recognized for who they truly are on a spiritual level, they will celebrate their existence. This is the essence of the Beloved on Earth and what it means to be –loved.

This frequency is associated with the absolute divine, the energy of Christ Consciousness. In this self-actualized state, you allow love to have its way with you, to run through you for the benefit of yourself and others. Breath by breath and minute by minute you return home. When you do so, everything in your life becomes beautiful because it is a reflection of your unique experience of God. Your house design, cooking, children, poetry, garden, photos, and clothing choices all begin to express the abundance of your inner experience. When you embody the divine feminine, you cultivate all the qualities that She emits. With increased multidimensional awareness, your creativity will expand and all of your life endeavors will be blessed. This allows others to experience the divine through your unique design, especially the creation of your children.

We all have this potential within, but it requires conscious intent and a genuine desire to vibrate in the world with this type of a frequency. As you know by now, it takes grace and grit to become clear enough to express the Beloved. My goal is for you to experience this at the time of conception and especially throughout your pregnancy. In order for this to happen, I am going to break down all the aspects of life that can affect wellness. In this chapter, I will review much of what we have covered throughout the book, and include some new insights, so that you leave with a clear plan on how to consciously proceed. This work is ongoing. You will feel prepared and ready to uplift yourself and your growing family throughout motherhood.

Programming the Eight Original Cells and Eight Aspects of Self

At the beginning of the book, I mentioned that there are eight original cells that can be found within everyone's body throughout their life. These cells or spheres are also referred to as the Egg of Life. Melchizedek's quote is worth repeating here: "Your entire physical existence is dependent upon your Egg of Life structure. Everything about you was created through the Egg of Life form, right down to the color of your eyes, the shape of your nose, how long your fingers are and everything else. It's all based on this one form." The energetics of these original eight cells make up your entire structure. The clearer these cells are energetically when your baby is formed, the closer the child will be to his or her original nature.

Spirit advised me that these eight original cells can be broken down into the eight aspects of self which include Body, Mind, Environment, Spirit, Community, Emotions, Finances, and Work. If you work on these eight aspects of yourself, you will create a wholeness and a balanced approach to life which will be reflected through your child's ongoing development. As I discuss these qualities through-out the chapter, visually connect each of these aspects back to eight spheres. Each sphere should represent one of the original eight cells of your child. If your life is in balance, it will be a lot easier to run an energy connected to the Beloved. As a result, your baby's eight original cells, or Egg of Life, will vibrate this frequency.

Utilize this chapter as an ongoing workbook to continually release density and connect yourself back to Source. This is your reference for all the hard work you have put into changing yourself in order to increase your fertility and alter your family forever. Below you will find descriptions of the eight aspects of self, also referred to as the eight dimensions of wellness, and questions to continually dive into as you move closer to motherhood. You can take your time answering these questions and return to this section of the book as often as you wish or feel the need to. Observe how your answers change when you look at the questions later. The process of awakening is constantly unfolding. As your consciousness increases, your answers will change. This is how self-improvement works and this is the power of loving oneself fiercely—a quality required for conscious motherhood.

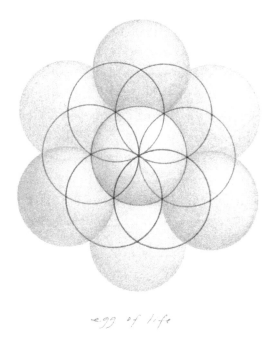

egg of life

Body: Recognize Your Physical Needs

Your body is a temple and it is also a vehicle to experiencing your best life on earth. The soul's essence is experienced through the body and is visually apparent within your physical appearance. Trauma and memories are all held within the physical form. When these experiences are not energetically released, they are passed down genetically to each generation. When someone is spiritually or mentally unwell, their physical body will display this energetic imbalance. If their heart is closed, the back may curve; a thyroid issue could possibly represent the inability to speak the truth; a person may look older than they truly are because the face displays mental constructs and worries. Paying attention to your body's physical attributes and level of wellness is important in the process of creating a healthy vessel for pregnancy. Focusing on your best qualities and gently healing the places where you still need to work on yourself will help you to thrive. Here are some important concepts to consider when it comes to raising the vibration of the physical body for conscious conception:

✣ Your body is a vehicle for experiencing the six senses and has the ability to let you feel the essence of each of these within your soul. Recall the last time you were in the ocean or a body of water. Did you really feel this experience on a cellular level or was your mind somewhere else when you were there? When you are in your body, you will embody experiences fully. In the ocean, you will feel the texture of the water, the sand beneath your feet, the wind blowing in your face, the fire of the sun beating down, and the essence of the higher realms through the clouds and birds around you. This is the full expression of divinity. When you experience the world around you like this when you are pregnant, you will program your baby to have the same type of presence within sacred experiences throughout life.

✣ Remember that your thoughts program your child. The way you view your physical body during pregnancy will affect your baby. Many women focus on the weight gain and have a difficult time adjusting to the physical changes their body goes through. As a result, they are energetically programming the baby in utero with the same self-deprecating thoughts. Be conscious of the way you speak about yourself and view your body so that your baby experiences self-love from the time in the womb and onward.

✣ Review the nutrition portion of this book and how to clear your genetic line. Is there anywhere that you could improve? Focus on adding one nutrient-dense food or energetically clearing one negative habit a week. This will have significant effects on yourself and your child.

✣ Consider your physical body the house for your baby. Every woman yearns to have her physical home prepared for her baby's arrival with a beautiful baby room that shows her outward devotion to creating life. How else can you prepare your physical body to hold a baby? Can you exercise more often? Add yoga to your routine or start dancing? Are there physical toxins to release? Just as you clear your house for spring cleaning, you must clear your body for the baby, letting go of anything that physically lowers your vibration.

✣ Anointing the body is an ancient ritual and form of self-love. How much self-care are you allowing? Are you holding tension within your body?

Consider asking your partner to massage you with an oil combined with two essential oil scents. Scents create an energetic signature for your baby at the time of conception, specifically when the cell splits in two to become the vesica piscis. What scents do you want to be associated with the creation of your child? Frankincense, myrrh, jasmine, lavender, sandalwood, and rose are a few examples.

Mind: Recognize Your Creative Abilities

I dedicated an entire chapter to the mind because it is one of the most powerful tools to improving your well-being during pregnancy. Here are some of the main takeaways from chapter five.

✤ As the screenwriter for an epic drama called "creating life," whatever you are thinking during pregnancy creates the dialogue for the movie that will play for your baby. The DNA of a baby can be affected in the womb by choosing positive thoughts and creating uplifting emotions.

✤ During the period of conception and pregnancy you must cultivate a mental picture of health and well-being. Higher frequency thoughts and feelings are based on love, harmony, acceptance, appreciation, trust, beauty, truth, peace, and reverence for God. If you aren't feeling well, or your emotions are negative, check what is on repeat in your mind. Do whatever is necessary to reverse these mental patterns.

✤ When you are pregnant, it is your perception of your environment and how you react to it that matters, not what is actually going on around you. Your mental projections and level of consciousness are what will be broadcast to your child. Even if you are in the midst of family chaos, you can actively choose to maintain images and feelings of love and harmony for your baby. The ultimate goal is to broadcast higher thoughts in order to maintain a peaceful vibration.

✤ The only way the fetus interprets the world is through the references of the mother. These are based on her mental projections and belief systems, which are predominately made up of subconscious programming from her own mother and childhood.

✦ The subconscious mind holds all your memories, events, patterns, and beliefs that you may not even know exist. When these are not released, they will overflow to other parts of our lives, creating neurosis, obsessions, depression, or negativity. When you are so full and heavy, you can't help but repeat the same mistakes, thought patterns or language throughout your life. This is why releasing negative thoughts, generational patterns, and belief systems is so important. It is also the reason you should start a meditation practice.

Environment: Create a Sacred Space

The womb is where the child is assembled and the environment of this space impacts the delicate assembly of the baby. Consider the environment or space around you to be a replica of the space that your child is growing in. What is the vibration of your surroundings and how can you create a sacred environment within and without? Can you alter your physical environment or your perception of it to create a more meditative experience for yourself and your child?

There are some family members and friends that are toxic. No matter how much work you do on yourself, after about thirty-six hours of being with them there are bound to be some subconscious triggers that arise. Sometimes this can happen within an hour. The time that you are pregnant is sacred; it is also relatively short within your lifespan. If you cannot maintain equilibrium while in the presence of certain people, my advice is to slip away from the situation. It is necessary to decide the exact type of environment you want to create when you are pregnant. Does it feel harmonious, loving, open, free of drama, and holy? Make a very clear intention for yourself of exactly the type of child you want to create and emulate that in your environment as much as possible.

Remember that your child is experiencing everything that you are experiencing. While your child is in the womb, imagine you are holding his or her hand and that both of you are going everywhere you are going and experiencing everything that you are experiencing. Every moment ask yourself, "Is this healthy for my child?"

Turn your life into a work of art. How can you make everything around you harmonious and beautiful? Can you enhance your environment through smells, colors, textures, paintings, sounds, altars, food, and heightened experiences? Is your life sacred?

Spirit: Expand the Meaning of Your Life

In *Mystical Motherhood*, I taught that it is necessary to meet basic needs before becoming a self-actualized individual. If you are living in survival mode, fear, or scarcity, it will be very difficult to fully connect to Spirit. These needs must be met in order to move up the ladder to full self-development and experience higher quality emotions such as love, belonging, high self-esteem and merging with God. Lower vibrational energies often cause a fight or flight response. This level of stress is detrimental to fertility and the creation of your child.

✤ There is a part of yourself that goes beyond all of the concepts spoken about here regarding environment, career or relationships. It is more powerful than any of those things. There is a part of you that is part of God. Can you connect to that part and can you perceive all the other aspects from this higher place? This is the place from which these higher children will experience the world and the place we should seek to parent them from.

✤ When you are stuck in the human drama and trauma, can you lift your soul up and experience yourself from higher point of view? This requires you to lift your energy above your body and peer down at the situation that you are in from above. When you do so, ask yourself, "Why did I choose these people and circumstances? What lessons do I still have to learn and how can I move through these earthly situations in order to raise my consciousness?"

✤ Letting go of the human story will alter your life. The human story is the repetition of all of the attachments we hold onto through perceived needs and fears which manifest through every aspect of life. This could be holding onto the same relationship patterns that can arise in various forms such as abuse, martyr syndrome, victimhood, manipulation or issues with dominance. Any attachment to the human form creates density. The more you can release physically, emotionally, mentally, and spiritually, the freer you become. As your consciousness expands, you become the gateway for more conscious Beings to come through you.

Community: Develop a Balanced Support System

One of the biggest influences on well-being, and even on longevity, is feeling a sense of fulfillment through community. An issue facing mothers today is lack of support and community after having their baby. In ancient times, women often planned their pregnancies and the community was involved in this as it impacted the whole unit. Women were taken care of for extended periods after birth, and groups of women bonded over sharing responsibilities for multiple children. Sadly, this is not the case in modern times and we are faced with increased isolation which causes a significant amount of depression in mothers.

* As much as we believe that social media is a resource for community, it does not create the same type of physical or social interaction that is required in motherhood. There are many social media communities for mothers that create inaccurate representations of what motherhood looks like. This in turn creates misinterpretations around birth, postpartum and child raising. Do not fully base your sense of community on online networks. Also, do not create belief systems of what pregnancy or motherhood should look like based on what anyone else is creating in their own reality. It may be necessary to stop following certain people or organizations that create any sense of unworthiness. Create your own unique interpretation of reality.

* In *Mystical Motherhood*, I went into greater detail about the importance of creating community, especially when you are postpartum. Build your community throughout pregnancy so that you have individuals or groups to reach out to when your baby arrives. If you are currently struggling with infertility, reach out to other women who have gone through this process so that you do not feel isolation around your journey. Feel free to write in to *Mystical Motherhood* for further support.

Emotions: An Energetic Frequency

Emotions are the key indicators of where our thoughts are at, and feelings are necessary in the process of awakening. Emotions can be used to guide us or they can destroy us if we are controlled by them. Avoiding pain and seeking pleasure are forms of spiritually bypassing all the work that needs to be done to free ourselves.

♣ You have a choice right now. You can allow your emotions to take you over or you can become consciously aware of how you act and react. You have the power to drop your problems. Use your emotions as a navigation system to determine your thoughts and current vibration.

♣ When you choose a better thought, you will also improve your emotions and overall energetic frequency. If you are stuck in negativity, play mantras—they help to switch the mind from negativity to positivity and rapidly increase your energy.

♣ Yogi Bhajan taught that women are sixteen times more intuitive than men or sixteen times more neurotic. The choice is up to you. The more you work on yourself, by creating a healthy lifestyle and meditative mind state, the easier it will be to manage your emotions.

♣ Moon Centers: An excellent way to understand the trajectory of your changing emotions is by mapping how your eleven moon centers move over the month. The moon centers are different from your monthly menstruation cycle and they change approximately every two and a half days. You cannot change how your emotions affect you as they move through your moon centers. You can, however, understand what moon center you are in so that you have a sincere respect for what you are feeling. When you know what moon center your energy is flowing through, you will become very powerful. Understanding your moon centers helps you to map your emotions. This will allow you to plan ahead and master your environment in subtle ways.

♣ Yogi Bhajan described the moon centers like this, "There are eleven sites of the moon on a woman, through which the moon moves in a 28-day cycle, spending two and a half days at each center. The sequence varies with each woman, and it does not coincide with her menstrual or zodiac moon cycle. It is different with each woman but the sequence remains constant in any individual woman except in the case of an emotional shock which does change it. It can be predicted and known only by observation. A woman can always feel it if she just concentrates with sensitivity. A man can also learn her cycles with sensitive observation. (The male's moon center is in the chin, just as is the woman's center, but because of his hair, there, he is steady and not as changeable as a woman.)"

⚜ Below are the eleven moon centers and their corresponding emotions. Mapping your moon cycles is a form of self-psychology and an excellent way to get to know your emotional well-being. Understand that it is subtle and knowing what center you are in comes through heightened intuition and a feeling of the center lighting up. You can ask yourself during meditation what center you are in by going through each area. You can also map your emotions and behaviors and then refer back to the descriptions below for guidance. Mapping your centers may take months.

Hairline   clarity and stability, nothing can move you, sensitive, magnetic, powerful, based in reality

Cheeks   unpredictability, out of control, go after people, see negativity, easily offended, a dangerous time

Lips   communication

Ear Lobes   demonstrate intelligence and ethics, affirm values

Back of Neck   romantic, flattered, easy to reach, etheric

Breasts   compassionate, over giving to the extent of foolishness

Navel   insecurity (the most sensitive time)

Inner Thighs   confirmative, defining, concrete

Eyebrows   imaginative, illusionary, artistic

Clitoris   talkative, eager to socialize

Vagina   depth and sharing

Finances: Abundance and Prosperity

Finance is spiritual abundance materialized in the physical world. Although many perceive financial success as acquisition of things from the outside to provide security, it is a lot more than this. Prosperity is a way of being when one is connected to their Source. It is also a natural human experience that is taken away by belief systems based on lack and scarcity which originate from the lower three chakras.

✤ Individuals who have a lot of money aren't usually the most abundant or prosperous people. Those who have accumulated a significant amount of physical cash often live with the greatest amount of fear, because they are constantly afraid of losing what they have. The experience of scarcity is created when the heart chakra is closed. Feeling that there is not enough is one of the most common misperceptions controlling the psyches of humans. Where in your life do you feel lack, or fear around not receiving? Where did these belief systems originate from in your history and how are they blocking your abundance?

✤ Success comes to those who know themselves and understand their connection to Source. When you trust in a higher power, there is always enough. You will be given exactly what you need when you need it. God gives to those who have an open mind and open heart. Work on your subconscious by clearing any fears you have around receiving or giving through meditation and you will see a vast amount of difference in how much you can create.

✤ Qualities of prosperity include truthfulness in your words, the feeling of security, grace in your actions and depth of your spirit. If you love to live, and experience life as a gift, you will truly understand what it means to be a wealthy person. One of the best ways to change your view towards abundance is to change your thoughts, and the words that you speak. Gratitude and enthusiasm for life are your greatest tools to creating more of what you want and need. Can you speak with these two experiences in mind and use words specific to these vibrations? Track the negative words that come out of your mouth regarding your self-worth and ability to create. How can you change your language to move through your blocks?

♣ The more you give, the more you will receive. People are often afraid that if they give away their money or time they will not have anything left. This is far from the truth. Those who are truly prosperous serve others. Like a flower, they open themselves up for the happiness of all.

♣ If you have felt in shock after giving something, you have likely been taken advantage of or have over given and not received. In these cases, giving happened faster than it should have. Some relationships are karmic and codependent, creating an unnatural balance. Examine all the relationships in your life. Is there balance in the giving and the taking? Are you in any codependent relationships that take away your power? How can you heal your relationship with giving in order to receive more?

♣ When you are living a truly abundant life, everything will come to you. You will no longer have to go out and chase after anything. You will realize that God is within you. This is the point of true creation. Your outside world reflects your internal experience. If you want abundance, financial security, and prosperity, work on yourself and create from there. Programming your child with this type of prosperity will change his or her destiny.

Work: Your Personal Satisfaction

One of the most common issues with my clients is a difficult working environment which impacts their stress level during the process of trying to conceive. Oftentimes it requires making boundaries or changing positions at work in order to reduce the cortisol or stress levels. This in turn requires a significant amount of letting go of control which is one of the biggest issues affecting fertility. The best thing to do is to change your perception of the environment, because there is an internal reason for every situation we are in. If you can't do this, and your job is negatively impacting your ability to function, you need to decide if this is the type of environment you would want to be in when you are pregnant. You also need to determine if this is the level of work you could handle with a child. How can you improve your current career?

✤ Changing careers to create more equilibrium may create an incredible amount of stress. If you leave your job for a new location because of negativity, it is likely that you will find yourself in a similar situation at some point. If you do not change your vibration you will naturally attract a similar frequency anywhere you go. This is the same as assuming a new relationship will be better if you find a new partner—the underlying problems will be carried over unless they are dealt with. Similar issues continuously arise in people and places until they are healed within you.

✤ I work with many clients to change their perception of the environment before they alter their career. This can be as simple as improving their office cubicle or looking at how the relationships with work colleagues mirror their own issues in need of healing. If a client is dealing with a controlling boss, we look at all the ways that this boss is showing her her own need to control.

✤ Your environment is critical during pregnancy. Sometimes changing your internal experience or perception of the situation is not enough. Energy vampires are real and they come in many forms. Certain individuals can suck your time, energy, emotions, and sense of well-being. The worst part about this is they thrive from doing so. If you have the luxury and possibility of removing yourself from an unbalanced situation that is causing you stress, then follow your intuition. If you feel you have done everything possible to heal a relationship or situation and it is still negative, walk away. Spirituality is not always "love and light," and boundaries are necessary. As your frequency changes, so will the people that are tolerable in your field. It is best to walk away from negativity before you become pregnant as you may find that doing so reduces your cortisol levels and improves your fertility.

The Path of the Holy Grail

Once you choose to become a reflection of your Cosmic Mother, she will do everything in her power to help you manifest what you want and need. In this case, your deepest desire is to create a child unlike any other. In your personal journey of awakening, you have humbly stepped into the role of assisting the awakening of humanity. There is a war going on within this planet, and the only way to change it is to be in your highest vibration. When you do this, you become a walking revolution. You have the power to end the fear, hate, disapproval, shame, guilt, pain, and depression that have run through your genetics for centuries. You are literally creating the Holy Grail within, and showing The Way for others.

Every great story returns to where it began, but you are now different. You experience the world through this new version of YOU. Picture yourself walking in your favorite place in nature again as I asked you to do at the beginning of the book. Do you have a different understanding of yourself and environment? Has your consciousness expanded to hold more within your auric field? Do you feel more connected to your mission of creating an enlightened soul for this planet? As a genetic engineer for humanity, you are the essence of the Cosmic Mother herself.

The feminine archetypes are reaching out to assist you in your endeavor. Call upon the Goddess, Ascended Masters, saints, sages, and angels on your journey through motherhood. In order to perform alchemy, you need a container, the substance you are transforming, and energy. This book has provided you with the tools to transform your body, mind, and spirit in order to become the sacred vessel capable of holding a high vibrational child. *Your mission is critical.* YOU are the womb which is the future. I commend your dedication to saving this planet through the service of motherhood. The power is now in your hands.

CPSIA information can be obtained
at www.ICGtesting.com
Printed in the USA
BVHW050749040122
625355BV00006BB/110